GLOBAL HEALTH RISKS

Mortality and burden of disease attributable to selected major risks

World Health Organization

WHO Library Cataloguing-in-Publication Data

Global health risks: mortality and burden of disease attributable to selected major risks.

1. Risk factors. 2. World health. 3. Epidemiology. 4. Risk assessment. 5. Mortality - trends. 6. Morbidity - trends. 7. Data analysis, Statistical. I. World Health Organization.

ISBN 978 92 4 156387 1
(NLM classification: WA 105)

© World Health Organization 2009

Acknowledgements

This publication was produced by the Department of Health Statistics and Informatics in the Information, Evidence and Research Cluster of the World Health Organization (WHO). The analyses were primarily carried out by Colin Mathers, Gretchen Stevens and Maya Mascarenhas, in collaboration with other WHO staff, WHO technical programmes and the Joint United Nations Programme on HIV/AIDS (UNAIDS). The report was written by Colin Mathers, Gretchen Stevens and Maya Mascarenhas.

We wish to particularly thank Majid Ezzati, Goodarz Danaei, Stephen Vander Hoorn, Steve Begg and Theo Vos for valuable advice and information relating to other international and national comparative risk assessment studies. Valuable inputs were provided by WHO staff from many departments and by experts outside WHO. Although it is not possible to name all those who contributed to this effort, we would like to particularly note the assistance and inputs provided by Bob Black, Ties Boerma, Sophie Bonjour, Fiona Bull, Diarmid Campbell-Lendrum, Mercedes de Onis, Regina Guthold, Mie Inoue, Doris Ma Fat, Annette Pruess, Jürgen Rehm, George Schmid and Petra Schuster.

Figures were prepared by Florence Rusciano, and design and layout were by Reto Schürch.

Contents

Tables

Figures

Summary

The leading global risks for mortality in the world are high blood pressure (responsible for 13% of deaths globally), tobacco use (9%), high blood glucose (6%), physical inactivity (6%), and overweight and obesity (5%). These risks are responsible for raising the risk of chronic diseases such as heart disease, diabetes and cancers. They affect countries across all income groups: high, middle and low.

The leading global risks for burden of disease as measured in disability-adjusted life years (DALYs) are underweight (6% of global DALYs) and unsafe sex (5%), followed by alcohol use (5%) and unsafe water, sanitation and hygiene (4%). Three of these risks particularly affect populations in low-income countries, especially in the regions of South-East Asia and sub-Saharan Africa. The fourth risk – alcohol use – shows a unique geographic and sex pattern, with its burden highest for men in Africa, in middle-income countries in the Americas and in some high-income countries.

This report uses a comprehensive framework for studying health risks developed for *The world health report 2002*, which presented estimates for the year 2000. The report provides an update for the year 2004 for 24 global risk factors. It uses updated information from WHO programmes and scientific studies for both exposure data and the causal associations of risk exposure to disease and injury outcomes. The burden of disease attributable to risk factors is measured in terms of lost years of healthy life using the metric of the disability-adjusted life year. The DALY combines years of life lost due to premature death with years of healthy life lost due to illness and disability.

Although there are many possible definitions of "health risk", it is defined in this report as "a factor that raises the probability of adverse health outcomes". The number of such factors is countless and the report does not attempt to be comprehensive. For example, some important risks associated with exposure to infectious disease agents or with antimicrobial resistance are not included. The report focuses on selected risk factors which have global spread, for which data are available to estimate population exposures or distributions, and for which the means to reduce them are known.

Five leading risk factors identified in this report (childhood underweight, unsafe sex, alcohol use, unsafe water and sanitation, and high blood pressure) are responsible for one quarter of all deaths in the world, and one fifth of all DALYs. Reducing exposure to these risk factors would increase global life expectancy by nearly 5 years.

Eight risk factors (alcohol use, tobacco use, high blood pressure, high body mass index, high cholesterol, high blood glucose, low fruit and vegetable intake, and physical inactivity) account for 61% of cardiovascular deaths. Combined, these same risk factors account for over three quarters of ischaemic heart disease: the leading cause of death worldwide. Although these major risk factors are usually associated with high-income countries, over 84% of the total global burden of disease they cause occurs in low- and middle-income countries. Reducing exposure to these eight risk factors would increase global life expectancy by almost 5 years.

A total of 10.4 million children died in 2004, mostly in low- and middle-income countries. An estimated 39% of these deaths (4.1 million) were caused by micronutrient deficiencies, underweight, suboptimal breastfeeding and preventable environmental risks. Most of these preventable deaths occurred in the WHO African Region (39%) and the South-East Asia Region (43%).

Nine environmental and behavioural risks, together with seven infectious causes, are responsible for 45% of cancer deaths worldwide. For specific cancers, the proportion is higher: for example, tobacco smoking alone causes 71% of lung cancer deaths worldwide. Tobacco accounted for 18% of deaths in high-income countries.

Health risks are in transition: populations are ageing owing to successes against infectious diseases; at the same time, patterns of physical activity and food, alcohol and tobacco consumption are changing. Low- and middle-income countries now face a double burden of increasing chronic, noncommunicable conditions, as well as the communicable diseases that traditionally affect the poor. Understanding the role of these risk factors is important for developing clear and effective strategies for improving global health.

Abbreviations

AIDS .... acquired immunodeficiency syndrome
BMI .... body mass index
CRA .... comparative risk assessment
DALY .... disability-adjusted life year
GBD .... global burden of disease
HIV .... human immunodeficiency virus
IUGR .... intrauterine growth restriction
MET .... metabolic equivalent (energy expenditure measured in units of resting energy expenditure)
PAF .... population attributable fraction
UNAIDS .... Joint United Nations Programme on HIV/AIDS
UNICEF .... United Nations Children's Fund
WHO .... World Health Organization
YLD .... years lost due to disability
YLL .... years of life lost (due to premature mortality)

1 Introduction

1.1 Purpose of this report

A description of diseases and injuries and the risk factors that cause them is vital for health decision-making and planning. Data on the health of populations and the risks they face are often fragmentary and sometimes inconsistent. A comprehensive framework is needed to pull together information and facilitate comparisons of the relative importance of health risks across different populations globally.

Most scientific and health resources go towards treatment. However, understanding the risks to health is key to preventing disease and injuries. A particular disease or injury is often caused by more than one risk factor, which means that multiple interventions are available to target each of these risks. For example, the infectious agent *Mycobacterium tuberculosis* is the direct cause of tuberculosis; however, crowded housing and poor nutrition also increase the risk, which presents multiple paths for preventing the disease. In turn, most risk factors are associated with more than one disease, and targeting those factors can reduce multiple causes of disease. For example, reducing smoking will result in fewer deaths and less disease from lung cancer, heart disease, stroke, chronic respiratory disease and other conditions. By quantifying the impact of risk factors on diseases, evidence-based choices can be made about the most effective interventions to improve global health.

This document – the *Global health risks* report – provides an update for the year 2004 of the comparative risk assessment (CRA) for 24 global risk factors. A comprehensive framework for studying health risks was previously published in the original CRA – referred to here as "CRA 2000" – which presented estimates for 22 global risk factors and their attributable estimates of deaths and burden of disease for the year 2000 *(1)*. This report uses updated information from WHO programmes and scientific studies for both exposure data and the causal associations of risk exposure to disease and injury outcomes. It applies these updated risk analyses to the latest regional estimates of mortality and disease burden for a comprehensive set of diseases and injuries for the year 2004 *(2)*.

1.2 Understanding the nature of health risks

To prevent disease and injury, it is necessary to identify and deal with their causes – the health risks that underlie them. Each risk has its own causes too, and many have their roots in a complex chain of events over time, consisting of socioeconomic factors, environmental and community conditions, and individual behaviour. The causal chain offers many entry points for intervention.

As can be seen from the example of ischaemic heart disease (**Figure 1**), some elements in the chain, such as high blood pressure or cholesterol, act as a relatively direct cause of the disease. Some risks located further back in the causal chain act indirectly through intermediary factors. These risks include physical inactivity, alcohol, smoking or fat intake. For the most distal risk factors, such as education and income, less causal certainty can be attributed to each risk. However, modifying these background causes is more likely to have amplifying effects, by influencing multiple proximal causes; such modifications therefore have the potential to yield fundamental and sustained improvements to health *(3)*.

In addition to multiple points of intervention along the causal chain, there are many ways that populations can be targeted. The two major approaches to reducing risk are:

- targeting high-risk people, who are most likely to benefit from the intervention
- targeting risk in the entire population, regardless of each individual's risk and potential benefit.

For example, a high-risk intervention for reducing high blood pressure would target the members of the population whose systolic blood pressure lies above 140 mmHg, which is considered hypertensive. However, a large proportion of the population are not considered to be hypertensive, but still have higher than ideal blood pressure levels and thus also face a raised health risk *(4)*. Although the risks for this group are lower than for those classified as hypertensive, there may be more deaths due to high blood pressure in this group because of the larger numbers of people it contains. Considering only the effect of hypertension on population health, as is often done, gives decision-makers an incomplete picture of the

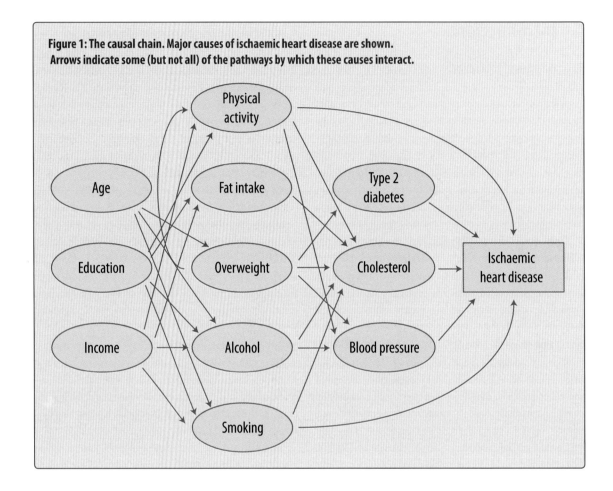

Figure 1: The causal chain. Major causes of ischaemic heart disease are shown. Arrows indicate some (but not all) of the pathways by which these causes interact.

importance of the risk factor for the population because it underestimates the full effect of raised blood pressure on population health. In this report, therefore, exposures are estimated across the entire population and are compared with an ideal scenario, rather than simply focusing on the group that is clinically at high risk.

Population-based strategies seek to change the social norm by encouraging an increase in healthy behaviour and a reduction in health risk. They target risks via legislation, tax, financial incentives, health-promotion campaigns or engineering solutions. However, although the potential gains are substantial, the challenges in changing these risks are great. Population-wide strategies involve shifting the responsibility of tackling big risks from individuals to governments and health ministries, thereby acknowledging that social and economic factors strongly contribute to disease.

1.3 The risk transition

As a country develops, the types of diseases that affect a population shift from primarily infectious, such as diarrhoea and pneumonia, to primarily non-communicable, such as cardiovascular disease and cancers (5). This shift is caused by:

- improvements in medical care, which mean that children no longer die from easily curable conditions such as diarrhoea
- the ageing of the population, because noncommunicable diseases affect older adults at the highest rates
- public health interventions such as vaccinations and the provision of clean water and sanitation, which reduce the incidence of infectious diseases.

This pattern can be observed across many countries, with wealthy countries further advanced along this transition.

Similarly, the risks that affect a population also shift over time, from those for infectious disease to those that increase noncommunicable disease (**Figure 2**). Low-income populations are most affected by risks associated with poverty, such as undernutrition, unsafe sex, unsafe water, poor sanitation and hygiene, and indoor smoke from solid fuels; these are the so-called "traditional risks". As life expectancies increase and the major causes of death and disability shift to the chronic and noncommunicable, populations are increasingly facing modern risks due to physical inactivity; overweight and obesity, and other diet-related factors; and tobacco and alcohol-related risks. As a result, many low- and middle-income countries now face a growing burden from the modern risks to health, while still fighting an unfinished battle with the traditional risks to health.

The impact of these modern risks varies at different levels of socioeconomic development. For example, urban air pollution is a greater risk factor in middle-income countries than in high-income countries because of substantial progress by the latter in controlling this risk through public-health policies (**Figure 2**). Increasing exposure to these emerging risks is not inevitable: it is amenable to public health intervention. For example, by enacting strong tobacco-control policies, low- and middle-income countries can learn from the tobacco-control successes in high-income countries. By enacting such policies early on, they can avoid the high levels of disease caused by tobacco currently found in high-income countries.

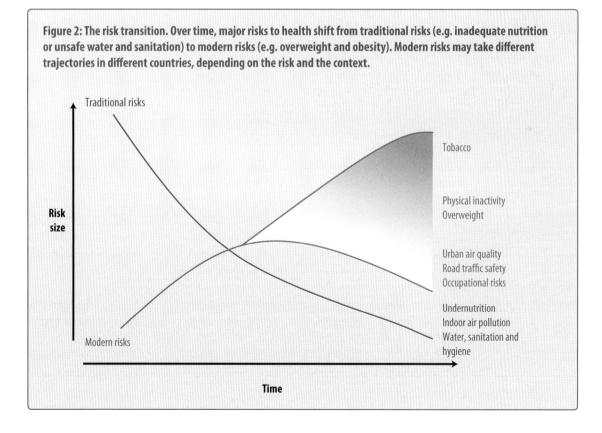

Figure 2: The risk transition. Over time, major risks to health shift from traditional risks (e.g. inadequate nutrition or unsafe water and sanitation) to modern risks (e.g. overweight and obesity). Modern risks may take different trajectories in different countries, depending on the risk and the context.

1.4 Measuring impact of risk

This report aims to systematically estimate the current burden of disease and injury in the world's population resulting from exposure to risks – known as the "attributable" burden of disease and injury. We calculate the attributable burden by estimating the population attributable fraction; that is, the proportional reduction in population disease or mortality that would occur if exposure to a risk factor were reduced to an alternative ideal exposure scenario (**Figure 3**). The number of deaths and DALYs (**see Box 1**) attributed to a risk factor is quantified by applying the population attributable fraction to the total number of deaths or the total burden of disease (see Annex A for calculation details). The burden of disease – measured in DALYs – quantifies the gap between a population's current health and an ideal situation where everyone lives to old age in full health.

For some risk factors, the ideal exposure level is clear; for example, zero tobacco use is the ideal. In other cases, the ideal level of exposure is less clear. As noted above, a large group of people fall within the clinically "normal" range for blood pressure (i.e. below 140 mmHg) but have blood pressure levels above ideal levels. We select ideal exposures that minimize risk to health. For blood pressure, this means selecting a blood pressure that is not only within the range considered normal, but is also at the low end of that range.

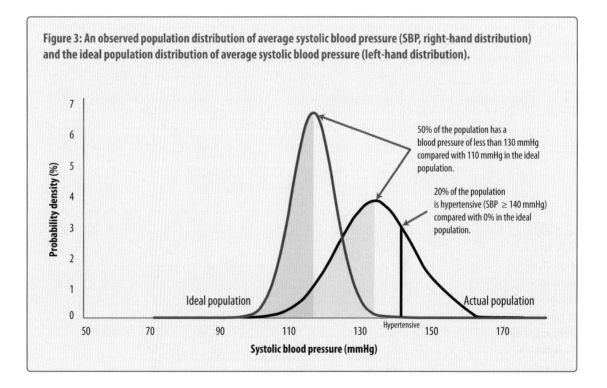

Figure 3: An observed population distribution of average systolic blood pressure (SBP, right-hand distribution) and the ideal population distribution of average systolic blood pressure (left-hand distribution).

> **Box 1: Disability-adjusted life years (DALYs)**
>
> DALYs are a common currency by which deaths at different ages and disability may be measured. One DALY can be thought of as one lost year of "healthy" life, and the burden of disease can be thought of as a measurement of the gap between current health status and an ideal situation where everyone lives into old age, free of disease and disability.
>
> DALYs for a disease or injury are calculated as the sum of the years of life lost due to premature mortality (YLL) in the population and the years lost due to disability (YLD) for incident cases of the disease or injury. YLL are calculated from the number of deaths at each age multiplied by a global standard life expectancy of the age at which death occurs. YLD for a particular cause in a particular time period are estimated as follows:
>
> YLD = number of incident cases in that period × average duration of the disease × disability weight
>
> The disability weight reflects the severity of the disease on a scale from 0 (perfect health) to 1 (death). The disability weights used for global burden of disease DALY estimates are listed elsewhere (6).
>
> In the standard DALYs in recent WHO reports, calculations of YLD used an additional 3% time discounting and non-uniform age weights that give less weight to years lived at young and older ages (7). Using discounting and age weights, a death in infancy corresponds to 33 DALYs, and deaths at ages 5–20 years to around 36 DALYs.

This report estimates how much burden of disease and injury for 2004 is attributable to 24 selected risk factors (counting the selected occupational risks as one risk factor). These environmental, behavioural and physiological risk factors were selected as having global spread, data available to estimate population exposures and outcomes, and potential for intervention. There are many other risks for health which are not included in the report. In particular, some important risk factors associated with infectious disease agents or with antimicrobial resistance are not included.

Many diseases are caused by multiple risk factors, and individual risk factors may interact in their impact on the overall risk of disease. As a result, attributable fractions of deaths and burden for individual risk factors usually overlap and often add up to more than 100%. For example, two risk factors – smoking and urban air pollution –cause lung cancer. As **Figure 4** below illustrates, some lung cancer deaths are attributed to more than one exposure – represented by the area where the circles overlap. This overlapping area represents the percentage of lung cancer deaths in 2004 that could have been averted if either tobacco exposure or urban air pollution had been lower.

The disease and injury outcomes caused by risk exposures are quantified in terms of deaths and DALYs for 2004, as described in a recently released WHO report (2). More-detailed tables of deaths and DALYs for disease and injury causes are available for a number of regional groupings of countries on the WHO web site.[1] **Box 2** provides an overview of the global burden of diseases and injuries.

1.5 Risk factors in the update for 2004

The risk factors chosen for this report all fulfil a number of criteria:

- a potential for a global impact
- a high likelihood that the risk causes each associated disease
- a potential for modification
- being neither too broad (e.g. diet) nor too specific (e.g. lack of broccoli)
- reasonably complete data were available for that risk.

This update for 2004 builds on the previous WHO CRA for the year 2000 (1). It does not include a complete review and revision of data inputs and

---

[1] http://www.who.int/evidence/bod

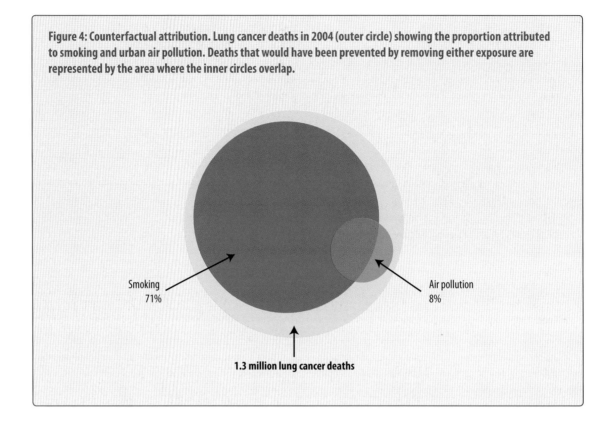

Figure 4: Counterfactual attribution. Lung cancer deaths in 2004 (outer circle) showing the proportion attributed to smoking and urban air pollution. Deaths that would have been prevented by removing either exposure are represented by the area where the inner circles overlap.

Smoking
71%

Air pollution
8%

1.3 million lung cancer deaths

estimates for every risk factor. The methods and data sources are described in detail in Annex A. The main changes in the 2004 estimates are as follows:

- Risk factor exposure estimates were revised if new estimates were available. For some risk factors (listed in Annex A), previously estimated population exposures were used.
- Where a recent peer-reviewed meta-analysis was available, relative risks from the 2000 CRA analysis were updated. Likewise, some minor revisions to methods based on peer-reviewed publications from WHO programmes or collaborating academic groups were incorporated and are explained in Annex A.
- Two additional risk factors have been included: suboptimal breastfeeding and high blood glucose, based on published peer-reviewed work (8, 9).

For all risk factors, some data were extrapolated when direct information was unavailable; direct information is often absent or scanty in developing countries, where the effects of many risks are highest. Perfect data on a health hazard's potential impact will never exist, so using such projections is justified. Nevertheless, it is important to treat estimates of numerical risk and its consequences with care.

The Bill & Melinda Gates Foundation is funding a study of the global burden of disease in 2005, which is due to be published in late 2010. The study is led by the Institute for Health Metrics and Evaluation at the University of Washington, with key collaborating institutions including WHO, Harvard University, Johns Hopkins University and the University of Queensland (10). The 2005 global burden of disease study will include a comprehensive revision and update of mortality and burden of disease attributable to an extended set of global risks. Where needed, major revisions of methods based on new evidence will be undertaken as part of this study.

1.6 Regional estimates for 2004

This report presents estimates for regional groupings of countries (including the six WHO regions) and income groupings, with the countries grouped as high, medium or low income, depending on their gross national income per capita in 2004. The classification of countries most commonly used here is seven groups, comprising the six WHO regions plus the high-income countries in all regions forming a seventh group (**Figure 5**). Lists of countries in each regional and income group are available in **Table A5** (**Annex A**). Detailed tables of results by cause, age, sex and region are available on the WHO web site[1] for a range of different regional groupings.

High-income countries represent 15% of the world population, middle-income countries about 47% and low-income countries about 37%. The distribution of deaths is similar to that of population across the country income groups, despite the comparatively young populations in the middle-income countries, and the even younger populations in the low-income countries. In contrast, more than half of DALYs occur in low-income countries. A further 38% occur in middle-income countries, while only 8% occur in high-income countries.

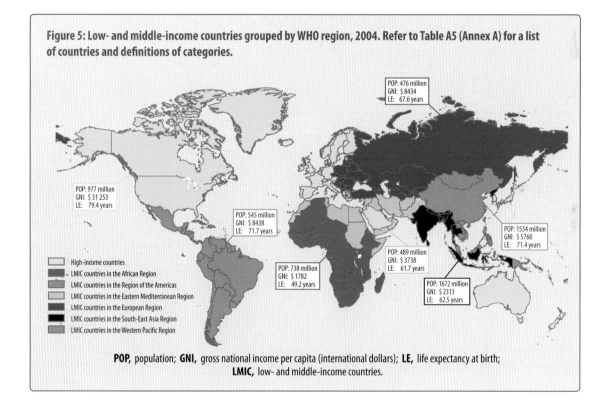

Figure 5: Low- and middle-income countries grouped by WHO region, 2004. Refer to Table A5 (Annex A) for a list of countries and definitions of categories.

POP: 476 million
GNI: $ 8434
LE: 67.6 years

POP: 977 million
GNI: $ 31 253
LE: 79.4 years

POP: 545 million
GNI: $ 8438
LE: 71.7 years

POP: 1534 million
GNI: $ 5760
LE: 71.4 years

POP: 489 million
GNI: $ 3738
LE: 61.7 years

POP: 738 million
GNI: $ 1782
LE: 49.2 years

POP: 1672 million
GNI: $ 2313
LE: 62.5 years

- High-income countries
- LMIC countries in the African Region
- LMIC countries in the Region of the Americas
- LMIC countries in the Eastern Mediterranean Region
- LMIC countries in the European Region
- LMIC countries in the South-East Asia Region
- LMIC countries in the Western Pacific Region

POP, population; **GNI,** gross national income per capita (international dollars); **LE,** life expectancy at birth; **LMIC,** low- and middle-income countries.

---

[1] http://www.who.int/evidence/bod

Box 2: The global burden of diseases and injuries

The global burden of disease 2004 update provides a comprehensive assessment of the causes of loss of health in the different regions of the world, drawing on extensive WHO databases and on information provided by Member States *(2)*. This consolidated study assesses the comparative importance of diseases and injuries in causing premature death, loss of health and disability in different populations: by age, sex and for a range of country groupings by geographic region or country income, or both. Results at country and regional level are also available on the WHO web site (http://www.who.int/evidence/bod).

The study contains details of the leading causes of death, disability and burden of disease in various regions, and detailed estimates for 135 disease and injury cause categories. Findings include the following:

- Worldwide, Africa accounts for 9 out of every 10 child deaths due to malaria, for 9 out of every 10 child deaths due to AIDS, and for half of the world's child deaths due to diarrhoeal disease and pneumonia.

- In low-income countries, the leading cause of death is pneumonia, followed by heart disease, diarrhoea, HIV/AIDS and stroke. In developed or high-income countries, the list is topped by heart disease, followed by stroke, lung cancer, pneumonia and asthma or bronchitis.

- Men between the ages of 15 and 60 years have much higher risks of dying than women in the same age category in every region of the world. This is mainly because of injuries, including violence and conflict, and higher levels of heart disease. The difference is most pronounced in Latin America, the Caribbean, the Middle East and Eastern Europe.

- Depression is the leading cause of years lost due to disability, the burden being 50% higher for females than males. In all income strata, alcohol dependence and problem use is among the 10 leading causes of disability.

2 Results

2.1 Global patterns of health risk

More than one third of the world's deaths can be attributed to a small number of risk factors. The 24 risk factors described in this report are responsible for 44% of global deaths and 34% of DALYs; the 10 leading risk factors account for 33% of deaths (see Section 3.2). Understanding the role of these risk factors is key to developing a clear and effective strategy for improving global health.

The five leading global risks for mortality in the world are high blood pressure, tobacco use, high blood glucose, physical inactivity, and overweight and obesity. They are responsible for raising the risk of chronic diseases, such as heart disease and cancers. They affect countries across all income groups: high, middle and low (Table 1 and Figure 6).

This report measures the burden of disease, or lost years of healthy life, using the DALY: a measure that gives more weight to non-fatal loss of health and deaths at younger ages (Box 1). The leading global risks for burden of disease in the world are underweight and unsafe sex, followed by alcohol use and unsafe water, sanitation and hygiene (Figure 7). Three of the four leading risks for DALYs – underweight, unsafe sex, and unsafe water, sanitation and hygiene – increase the number and severity of new cases of infectious diseases, and particularly affect populations in low-income countries, especially in the regions of South-East Asia and sub-Saharan Africa (Table 2). Alcohol use has a unique geographic and sex pattern: it exacts the largest toll on men in Africa, in middle-income countries in the Americas, and in some high-income countries.

Geographical patterns

Substantially different disease patterns exist between high-, middle- and low-income countries. For high- and middle-income countries, the most important risk factors are those associated with chronic diseases such as heart diseases and cancer. Tobacco is one of the leading risks for both: accounting for 11% of the disease burden and 18% of deaths in high-income countries. For high-income countries,

alcohol, overweight and blood pressure are also leading causes of healthy life years lost: each being responsible for 6–7% of the total. In middle-income countries, risks for chronic diseases also cause the largest share of deaths and DALYs, although risks such as unsafe sex and unsafe water and sanitation also cause a larger share of burden of disease than in high-income countries (Tables 1 and 2).

In low-income countries, relatively few risks are responsible for a large percentage of the high number of deaths and loss of healthy years. These risks generally act by increasing the incidence or severity of infectious diseases. The leading risk factor for low-income countries is underweight, which represents about 10% of the total disease burden. In combination, childhood underweight, micronutrient deficiencies (iron, vitamin A and zinc) and suboptimal breastfeeding cause 7% of deaths and 10% of total disease burden. The combined burden from these nutritional risks is almost equivalent to the entire disease and injury burden of high-income countries.

Demographic patterns

The profile of risk changes considerably by age. Some risks affect children almost exclusively: underweight, undernutrition (apart from iron deficiency), unsafe water, smoke from household use of solid fuels and climate change. Few of the risk factors examined in this report affect adolescent health per se, although risk behaviours starting in adolescence do have a considerable effect on health at later ages. For adults, there are considerable differences depending on age. Most of the health burden from addictive substances, unsafe sex, lack of contraception, iron deficiency and child sex abuse occurs in younger adults. Most of the health burden from risk factors for chronic diseases such as cardiovascular disease and cancers occurs at older adult ages.

Men and women are affected about equally from risks associated with diet, the environment and unsafe sex. Men suffer more than 75% of the burden from addictive substances and most of the burden from occupational risks. Women suffer all of the burden from lack of contraception, 80% of the deaths caused by iron deficiency, and about two thirds of the burden caused by child sexual abuse.

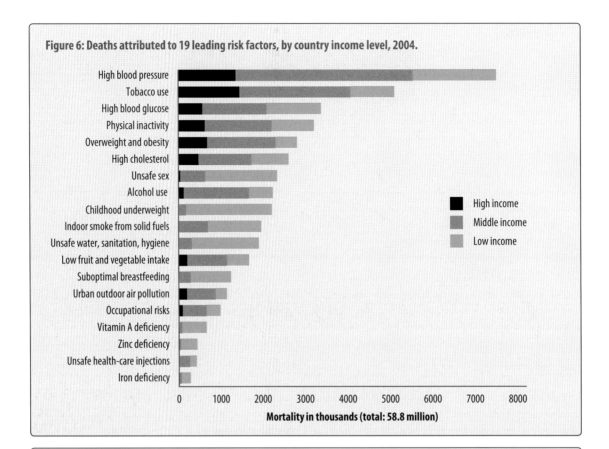

Figure 6: Deaths attributed to 19 leading risk factors, by country income level, 2004.

High blood pressure
Tobacco use
High blood glucose
Physical inactivity
Overweight and obesity
High cholesterol
Unsafe sex
Alcohol use
Childhood underweight
Indoor smoke from solid fuels
Unsafe water, sanitation, hygiene
Low fruit and vegetable intake
Suboptimal breastfeeding
Urban outdoor air pollution
Occupational risks
Vitamin A deficiency
Zinc deficiency
Unsafe health-care injections
Iron deficiency

High income
Middle income
Low income

Mortality in thousands (total: 58.8 million)

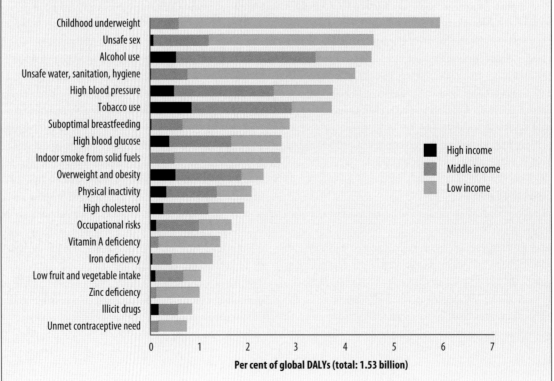

Figure 7: Percentage of disability-adjusted life years (DALYs) attributed to 19 leading risk factors, by country income level, 2004.

Childhood underweight
Unsafe sex
Alcohol use
Unsafe water, sanitation, hygiene
High blood pressure
Tobacco use
Suboptimal breastfeeding
High blood glucose
Indoor smoke from solid fuels
Overweight and obesity
Physical inactivity
High cholesterol
Occupational risks
Vitamin A deficiency
Iron deficiency
Low fruit and vegetable intake
Zinc deficiency
Illicit drugs
Unmet contraceptive need

High income
Middle income
Low income

Per cent of global DALYs (total: 1.53 billion)

Table 1: Ranking of selected risk factors: 10 leading risk factor causes of death by income group, 2004

	Risk factor	Deaths (millions)	Percentage of total		Risk factor	Deaths (millions)	Percentage of total
	World				*Low-income countries[a]*		
1	High blood pressure	7.5	12.8	1	Childhood underweight	2.0	7.8
2	Tobacco use	5.1	8.7	2	High blood pressure	2.0	7.5
3	High blood glucose	3.4	5.8	3	Unsafe sex	1.7	6.6
4	Physical inactivity	3.2	5.5	4	Unsafe water, sanitation, hygiene	1.6	6.1
5	Overweight and obesity	2.8	4.8	5	High blood glucose	1.3	4.9
6	High cholesterol	2.6	4.5	6	Indoor smoke from solid fuels	1.3	4.8
7	Unsafe sex	2.4	4.0	7	Tobacco use	1.0	3.9
8	Alcohol use	2.3	3.8	8	Physical inactivity	1.0	3.8
9	Childhood underweight	2.2	3.8	9	Suboptimal breastfeeding	1.0	3.7
10	Indoor smoke from solid fuels	2.0	3.3	10	High cholesterol	0.9	3.4
	Middle-income countries[a]				*High-income countries[a]*		
1	High blood pressure	4.2	17.2	1	Tobacco use	1.5	17.9
2	Tobacco use	2.6	10.8	2	High blood pressure	1.4	16.8
3	Overweight and obesity	1.6	6.7	3	Overweight and obesity	0.7	8.4
4	Physical inactivity	1.6	6.6	4	Physical inactivity	0.6	7.7
5	Alcohol use	1.6	6.4	5	High blood glucose	0.6	7.0
6	High blood glucose	1.5	6.3	6	High cholesterol	0.5	5.8
7	High cholesterol	1.3	5.2	7	Low fruit and vegetable intake	0.2	2.5
8	Low fruit and vegetable intake	0.9	3.9	8	Urban outdoor air pollution	0.2	2.5
9	Indoor smoke from solid fuels	0.7	2.8	9	Alcohol use	0.1	1.6
10	Urban outdoor air pollution	0.7	2.8	10	Occupational risks	0.1	1.1

[a] Countries grouped by gross national income per capita – low income (US$ 825 or less), high income (US$ 10 066 or more).

1

2

3

Annex A

References

Table 2: Ranking of selected risk factors: 10 leading risk factor causes of DALYs by income group, 2004

	Risk factor	DALYs (millions)	Percentage of total		Risk factor	DALYs (millions)	Percentage of total
	World				*Low-income countries[a]*		
1	Childhood underweight	91	5.9	1	Childhood underweight	82	9.9
2	Unsafe sex	70	4.6	2	Unsafe water, sanitation, hygiene	53	6.3
3	Alcohol use	69	4.5	3	Unsafe sex	52	6.2
4	Unsafe water, sanitation, hygiene	64	4.2	4	Suboptimal breastfeeding	34	4.1
5	High blood pressure	57	3.7	5	Indoor smoke from solid fuels	33	4.0
6	Tobacco use	57	3.7	6	Vitamin A deficiency	20	2.4
7	Suboptimal breastfeeding	44	2.9	7	High blood pressure	18	2.2
8	High blood glucose	41	2.7	8	Alcohol use	18	2.1
9	Indoor smoke from solid fuels	41	2.7	9	High blood glucose	16	1.9
10	Overweight and obesity	36	2.3	10	Zinc deficiency	14	1.7
	Middle-income countries[a]				*High-income countries[a]*		
1	Alcohol use	44	7.6	1	Tobacco use	13	10.7
2	High blood pressure	31	5.4	2	Alcohol use	8	6.7
3	Tobacco use	31	5.4	3	Overweight and obesity	8	6.5
4	Overweight and obesity	21	3.6	4	High blood pressure	7	6.1
5	High blood glucose	20	3.4	5	High blood glucose	6	4.9
6	Unsafe sex	17	3.0	6	Physical inactivity	5	4.1
7	Physical inactivity	16	2.7	7	High cholesterol	4	3.4
8	High cholesterol	14	2.5	8	Illicit drugs	3	2.1
9	Occupational risks	14	2.3	9	Occupational risks	2	1.5
10	Unsafe water, sanitation, hygiene	11	2.0	10	Low fruit and vegetable intake	2	1.3

[a] Countries grouped by 2004 gross national income per capita – low income (US$ 825 or less), high income (US$ 10 066 or more).

2.2 Childhood and maternal undernutrition

In low-income countries, easy-to-remedy nutritional deficiencies prevent 1 in 38 newborns from reaching age 5.

Many people in low- and middle-income countries, particularly children, continue to suffer from undernutrition[1]. They consume insufficient protein and energy, and the adverse health effects of this are often compounded by deficiencies of vitamins and minerals, particularly iodine, iron, vitamin A and zinc. Insufficient breast milk also puts infants at an increased risk of disease and death.

Of the risk factors quantified in this report, underweight is the largest cause of deaths and DALYs in children under 5 years, followed by suboptimal breastfeeding (Table 3). These and the other nutrition risks often coexist and contribute to the same disease outcomes. Because of overlapping effects, these risk factors were together responsible for an estimated 3.9 million deaths (35% of total deaths) and 144 million DALYs (33% of total DALYs) in children less than 5 years old. The combined contribution of these risk factors to specific causes of death is highest for diarrhoeal diseases (73%), and close to 50% for pneumonia, measles and severe neonatal infections (Figure 8).

Other important vitamin and mineral deficiencies not quantified in this report include those for calcium, folate, vitamin B$_{12}$ and vitamin D. Calcium and vitamin D deficiency are important causes of rickets and poor bone mineralization in children. Maternal folate insufficiency increases the risk of some birth defects and other adverse pregnancy outcomes. Maternal B vitamin deficiencies may also be associated with adverse pregnancy outcomes and development disabilities in infants.

Underweight

Underweight mainly arises from inadequate diet and frequent infection, leading to insufficient intake of calories, protein, vitamins and minerals. Children under 5 years, and especially those aged 6 months to 2 years, are at particular risk. In 2004, about 20% (112 million) of children under 5 years were underweight (more than two standard deviations below the WHO Child Growth Standards median weight-for-age) in

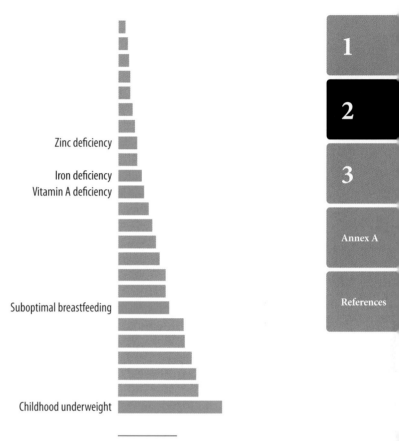

Zinc deficiency

Iron deficiency
Vitamin A deficiency

Suboptimal breastfeeding

Childhood underweight

See footnote 1

developing countries (see Annex A for details).

Underweight children suffer more frequent and severe infectious illnesses; furthermore, even mild undernutrition increases a child's risk of dying. Chronic undernutrition in children aged 24–36 months can also lead to long-term developmental problems; in adolescents and adults it is associated with adverse pregnancy outcomes and reduced ability to work. Around one third of diarrhoea, measles, malaria and lower respiratory infections in childhood are attributable to underweight. Of the 2.2 million child deaths attributable to underweight globally in 2004, almost half, or 1.0 million, occurred in the WHO African Region, and more than 800 000 in the South-East Asia Region.

Iron deficiency

Iron is critically important in muscle, brain and red blood cells. Iron deficiency may occur at any age if diets are based on staple foods with little meat, or people are exposed to infections that cause blood

---

[1] The schematic shows where the health burden of risk factors in this section fall in comparison to other risks in this report. It is repeated in each section; the full values can be found in Table A4.

Table 3: Deaths and DALYs attributable to six risk factors for child and maternal undernutrition, and to six risks combined; countries grouped by income, 2004

Risk	World	Low income	Middle income
Percentage of deaths			
Childhood underweight	3.8	7.8	0.7
Suboptimal breastfeeding	2.1	3.7	1.1
Vitamin A deficiency	1.1	2.2	0.3
Zinc deficiency	0.7	1.5	0.2
Iron deficiency	0.5	0.8	0.2
Iodine deficiency	0.0	0.0	0.0
All six risks	**6.6**	**12.7**	**2.1**
Percentage of DALYs			
Childhood underweight	6.0	9.9	1.5
Suboptimal breastfeeding	2.9	4.1	1.7
Vitamin A deficiency	1.5	2.4	0.4
Zinc deficiency	1.0	1.7	0.3
Iron deficiency	1.3	1.6	1.0
Iodine deficiency	0.2	0.2	0.3
All six risks	**10.4**	**15.9**	**4.4**

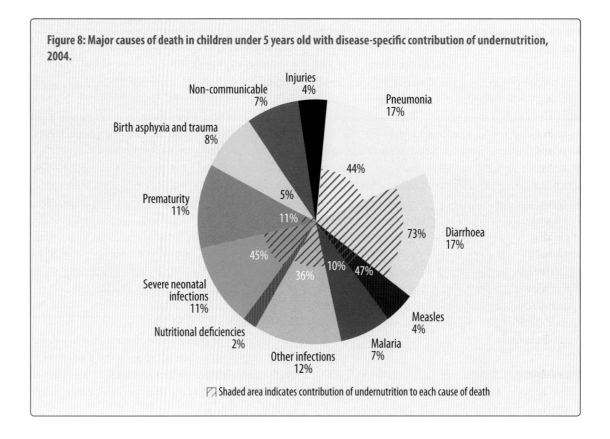

Figure 8: Major causes of death in children under 5 years old with disease-specific contribution of undernutrition, 2004.

Injuries 4%
Non-communicable 7%
Pneumonia 17%
Birth asphyxia and trauma 8%
44%
Prematurity 11%
5%
11%
73%
Diarrhoea 17%
45%
10% 47%
36%
Severe neonatal infections 11%
Measles 4%
Nutritional deficiencies 2%
Malaria 7%
Other infections 12%

Shaded area indicates contribution of undernutrition to each cause of death loss; young children and women of childbearing age are most commonly and severely affected. An estimated 41% of pregnant women and 27% of preschool children worldwide have anaemia caused by iron deficiency *(11)*.

Iron deficiency anaemia in early childhood reduces intelligence in mid-childhood; it can also lead to developmental delays and disability. About 18% of maternal mortality in low- and middle-income countries – almost 120 000 deaths – is attributable to iron deficiency. Adding this disease burden to that for iron deficiency anaemia in children and adults results in 19.7 million DALYs, or 1.3% of global total DALYs. Forty per cent of the total attributable global burden of iron deficiency occurs in the South-East Asia Region and almost another quarter in the African Region.

Vitamin A deficiency

Vitamin A is essential for healthy eyes, growth, immune function and survival. Deficiency is caused by low dietary intake, malabsorption and increased excretion due to common illnesses. It is the leading cause of acquired blindness in children. Those under 5 years and women of childbearing age are at most risk. About 33% of children suffer vitamin A deficiency (serum retinol <0.70 μmol/l), mostly in South-East Asia and Africa. The prevalence of low serum retinol is about 44% in African children and reaches almost 50% in children in South-East Asia *(12)*. The prevalence of night blindness caused by vitamin A deficiency is around 2% in African children, and about 0.5% in children in parts of South-East Asia. About 10% of women in Africa and South-East Asia experience night blindness during pregnancy.

Vitamin A deficiency raises the risk of mortality in children suffering from diarrhoeal diseases: 19% of global diarrhoea mortality can be attributed to this deficiency. It also increases the risk of mortality due to measles, prematurity and neonatal infections. Vitamin A deficiency is responsible for close to 6% of child deaths under age 5 years in Africa and 8% in South-East Asia.

Iodine deficiency

Iodine is essential for thyroid function. Iodine deficiency is one of the most easily preventable causes of mental retardation and developmental disability. Maternal iodine deficiency has also been associated with lower mean birth weight, increased infant mortality, impaired hearing and motor skills.

Although salt iodization and iodine supplementation programmes have reduced the number of countries where iodine deficiency remains a problem, about 1.9 billion people – 31% of the world population – do not consume enough iodine. The most affected WHO regions are South-East Asia and Europe *(13)*. The direct sequelae of iodine deficiency, such as goitre, cretinism and developmental disability, resulted in 3.5 million DALYs (0.2% of the total) in 2004.

Zinc deficiency

Zinc deficiency largely arises from inadequate intake or absorption from the diet, although diarrhoea may contribute. It increases the risk of diarrhoea, malaria and pneumonia, and is highest in South-East Asia and Africa *(9)*. For children under 5 years, zinc deficiency is estimated to be responsible for 13% of lower respiratory tract infections (mainly pneumonia and influenza), 10% of malaria episodes and 8% of diarrhoea episodes worldwide.

Suboptimal breastfeeding

Breast milk is the healthiest source of nutrition for infants. WHO recommends that infants should be exclusively breastfed during their first 6 months, and continue to receive breast milk through their first 2 years. In developing countries, only 24–32% of infants are exclusively breastfed at 6 months on average, and these percentages are much lower in developed countries. Rates of any breastfeeding are much higher, particularly in Africa and South-East Asia, with over 90% of infants aged 6–11 months breastfed.

Breastfeeding reduces the risk of many perinatal infections, acute lower respiratory infections and diarrhoea in infants below 23 months. Despite the higher prevalence of breastfeeding found in the developing world, developing countries bear more than 99% of the burden of suboptimal breastfeeding. Suboptimal breastfeeding is responsible for 45% of neonatal infectious deaths, 30% of diarrhoeal deaths and 18% of acute respiratory deaths in children under 5 years.

2.3 Other diet-related risk factors and physical inactivity

Worldwide, overweight and obesity cause more deaths than underweight.
The combined burden of these diet-related risks and physical inactivity in low- and middle-income countries is similar to that caused by HIV/AIDS and tuberculosis.

Over time, the risks that populations face tend to shift from risks (such as undernutrition) for infectious disease to risks for chronic disease, many of which are discussed in this section. This is because of past successes combating infectious diseases and their risks, and because populations worldwide are ageing, and these risk factors are more important for adults. Today, 65% of the world's population live in a country where overweight and obesity kills more people than underweight (this includes all high-income and most middle-income countries). The six risk factors discussed in this section account for 19% of global deaths and 7% of global DALYs. These risk factors have the greatest effect on cardiovascular diseases – 57% of cardiovascular deaths can be traced back to one of these risk factors. High blood pressure, which itself is caused by high body mass index (BMI) and physical inactivity, is the leading risk factor in this group (**Table 4**).

The DALYs lost per 10 000 population due to high cholesterol, high body mass index, high blood pressure, and all six risk factors combined are shown in **Figure 9** for high-income countries and for low- and middle-income countries grouped by WHO region. In all regions other than the Western Pacific, the low- and middle-income populations lose more DALYs because of these risks than populations in high-income countries. The attributable burden of disease per capita is greatest in the low- and middle-income countries of Europe.

High blood pressure
Raised blood pressure changes the structure of the arteries. As a result, risks of stroke, heart disease, kidney failure and other diseases increase, not only in people with hypertension but also in those with average, or even below-average, blood pressure. Diet – especially too much salt – alcohol, lack of exercise and obesity all raise blood pressure, and these effects

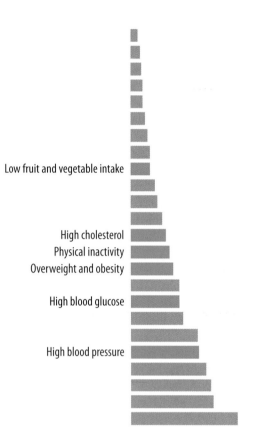

Low fruit and vegetable intake

High cholesterol
Physical inactivity
Overweight and obesity

High blood glucose

High blood pressure

accumulate with age. In developing and developed countries, most adults' blood pressure is higher than the ideal level. Average blood pressure levels are particularly high in middle-income European countries and African countries.

Globally, 51% of stroke (cerebrovascular disease) and 45% of ischaemic heart disease deaths are attributable to high systolic blood pressure. At any given age, the risk of dying from high blood pressure in low- and middle-income countries is more than double that in high-income countries. In the high-income countries, only 7% of deaths caused by high blood pressure occur under age 60; in the African Region, this increases to 25%.

High cholesterol
Diets high in saturated fat, physical inactivity and genetics can increase cholesterol levels. Recent research shows that levels of low-density lipoproteins and high-density lipoproteins are more important for health than total cholesterol. Nevertheless, we calculated the risk of elevated total blood cholesterol because there is more information available

Table 4: Deaths and DALYs attributable to six diet-related risks and physical inactivity, and to all six risks combined, by region, 2004

Risk	World	Low and middle income	High income
Percentage of deaths			
High blood pressure	12.8	12.1	16.8
High blood glucose	5.8	5.6	7.0
Physical inactivity	5.5	5.1	7.7
Overweight and obesity	4.8	4.2	8.4
High cholesterol	4.5	4.3	5.8
Low fruit and vegetable intake	2.9	2.9	2.5
All six risks	19.1	18.1	25.2
Percentage of DALYs			
High blood pressure	3.8	3.5	6.1
High blood glucose	2.7	2.5	4.9
Physical inactivity	2.1	1.9	4.1
Overweight and obesity	2.4	2.0	6.5
High cholesterol	2.0	1.8	3.4
Low fruit and vegetable intake	1.1	1.0	1.3
All six risks	7.0	6.5	12.6

about average total cholesterol levels in populations worldwide than about average low-density lipoproteins and high-density lipoprotein levels.

Cholesterol increases the risks of heart disease, stroke and other vascular diseases. Globally, one third of ischaemic heart disease is attributable to high blood cholesterol. High blood cholesterol increases the risk of heart disease, most in the middle-income European countries, and least in the low- and middle-income countries in Asia.

High blood glucose

Changes in diet and reductions in physical inactivity levels increase resistance to insulin, which, in turn, raises blood glucose. Genetics play an important role in whether individuals with similar diets and physical activity levels become resistant to insulin. Individuals with high levels of insulin resistance are classified as having diabetes, but individuals with raised blood glucose who do not have diabetes also face higher risks of cardiovascular diseases.

Globally, 6% of deaths are caused by high blood glucose, with 83% of those deaths occurring in low- and middle-income countries. The age-specific risk of dying from high blood glucose is lowest in high-income countries and the WHO Western Pacific Region. Raised blood glucose causes all diabetes deaths, 22% of ischaemic heart disease and 16% of stroke deaths.

Overweight and obesity (high body mass index)

WHO estimates that, in 2005, more than 1 billion people worldwide were overweight (BMI ≥ 25) and more than 300 million were obese (BMI ≥ 30). Mean BMI, overweight and obesity are increasing worldwide due to changes in diet and increasing physical inactivity. Rates of overweight and obesity are projected to increase in almost all countries, with 1.5 billion people overweight in 2015 *(14)*. Average BMI is highest in the Americas, Europe and the Eastern Mediterranean.

The risk of coronary heart disease, ischaemic stroke and type 2 diabetes grows steadily with increasing body mass, as do the risks of cancers of the breast, colon, prostate and other organs. Chronic overweight contributes to osteoarthritis – a major cause of disability. Globally, 44% of diabetes burden, 23% of ischaemic heart disease burden and 7–41% of certain cancer burdens are attributable to overweight and obesity. In both South-East Asia and Africa, 41% of deaths caused by high body mass index occur under age 60, compared with 18% in high-income countries.

Low fruit and vegetable intake

Fruit and vegetable consumption is one element of a healthy diet *(15, 16)*. Fruit and vegetable intake varies considerably among countries: reflecting economic, cultural and agricultural environments.

Insufficient intake of fruit and vegetables is estimated to cause around 14% of gastrointestinal cancer deaths, about 11% of ischaemic heart disease deaths and about 9% of stroke deaths worldwide. Most of the benefit of consuming fruits and vegetables comes from reduction in cardiovascular disease,

but fruits and vegetables also prevent cancer. Rates of deaths and DALYs attributed to low fruit and vegetable intake are highest in middle-income European countries and in South-East Asia.

Physical inactivity

Physical activity reduces the risk of cardiovascular disease, some cancers and type 2 diabetes. It can also improve musculoskeletal health, control body weight and reduce symptoms of depression. Physical activity occurs across different domains, including work, transport, domestic duties and during leisure. In high-income countries, most activity occurs during leisure time, while in low-income countries most activity occurs during work, chores or transport. Physical inactivity is estimated to cause around 21–25% of breast and colon cancer burden, 27% of diabetes and about 30% of ischaemic heart disease burden.

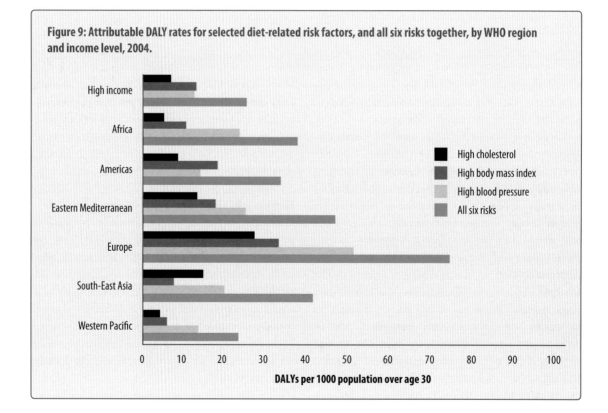

Figure 9: Attributable DALY rates for selected diet-related risk factors, and all six risks together, by WHO region and income level, 2004.

2.4   Sexual and reproductive health

Unsafe sex is the leading risk factor for mortality in African women: 1 million African women are killed annually by HIV, human papillomavirus and other sexually transmitted infections.

We consider sexual behaviours that increase the risk of contracting a sexually transmitted disease as a risk factor – "unsafe sex" – separate from the risk of unintended pregnancy, and its health consequences, associated with non-use and use of ineffective methods of contraception. Using certain forms of contraception, such as condoms, reduces both these risks, but other forms of risk reduction are quite different. Other factors involved in reducing unsafe sex include number of partners, who the partners are, the type of sex involved, knowledge of infection status of partners and use of barrier contraceptives.

Unsafe sex

People's sexual behaviour varies greatly between countries and regions. In 2004, unsafe sex was estimated as being responsible for more than 99% of human immunodeficiency virus (HIV) infection in Africa – the only region where more women than men are infected with HIV or acquired immunodeficiency syndrome (AIDS). Elsewhere, the proportion of HIV/AIDS deaths due to unsafe sex ranges from around 50% in the low- and middle-income countries of the WHO Western Pacific Region to 90% in the low- and middle-income countries of the Americas. In virtually all regions outside Africa, HIV transmission due to unsafe sex occurs predominantly among sex workers and men who have sex with men.

HIV/AIDS is the world's sixth biggest cause of death, and was responsible for 2.0 million deaths in 2004. HIV/AIDS deaths have stabilized and begun to decline in the last few years, partly due to increasing access to HIV treatment and also partly because of changing patterns of sexual behaviour in heavily affected African countries. Currently, 22 million (67%) of the 33 million people with HIV live in Africa, and HIV/AIDS continues to have a heavy impact: life expectancy at birth in the African Region was 49 years in 2004 (without AIDS it would have been 53 years).

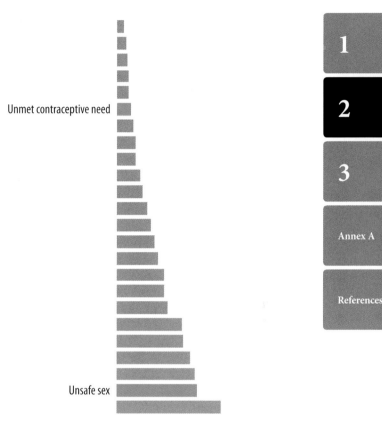

All cervical cancer is attributed to sexual transmission of the human papillomavirus. Cervical cancer accounts for 11% of global deaths due to unsafe sex, and is the leading cause of cancer death in the African Region. Almost three quarters of the global burden of unsafe sex occurs in sub-Saharan Africa, and another 15% in India and other countries of the South-East Asia Region. Other sexually transmitted infections such as syphilis, gonorrhoea and chlamydia are entirely attributable to unsafe sex.

Lack of contraception

Non-use and use of ineffective methods of contraception increase the risk of unintended pregnancy and its consequences, including unsafe abortions. The proportion of women aged 15–44 years who used modern contraception (such as the pill, barrier methods, sterilization or intrauterine device) ranged from 14% in the WHO African Region to 64% in high-income countries. If all women who wanted to space or limit future pregnancies used modern methods, usage would range from 46% in the African Region to 83% in the low- and middle-income countries of the Americas.

Unintended pregnancy leads to unwanted and mistimed births, with the same maternal and perinatal complications as planned births. The risk of abortion-related complications is proportional to the risk of unsafe abortion, which is strongly related to the legality of abortion in the country concerned. Unplanned pregnancies are estimated to be responsible for 30% of the disease burden associated with maternal conditions and around 90% of unsafe abortions globally.

Globally, lack of modern contraception caused around 0.3% of deaths and 0.8% of DALYs. Africa, South-East Asia and low- and middle-income countries in the Eastern Mediterranean Region had the highest disease burden due to lack of contraception – accounting for around 0.5% of deaths and 1.0– 1.2% of DALYs in those regions (**Figure 10**).

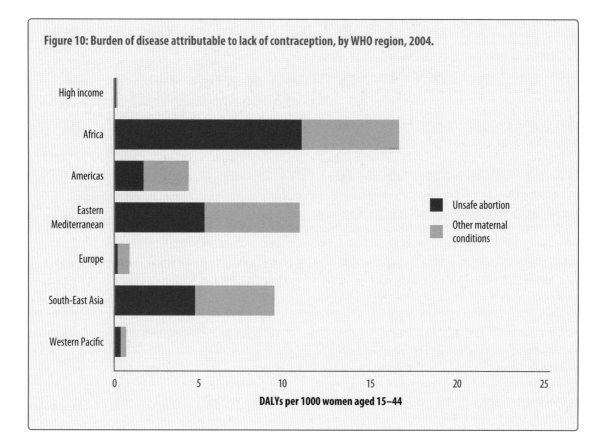

Figure 10: Burden of disease attributable to lack of contraception, by WHO region, 2004.

2.5 Addictive substances

In 2004, 70% of deaths caused by tobacco use occurred in low- and middle-income countries.

Smoking and oral tobacco use

Smoking substantially increases the risk of death from lung and other cancers, heart disease, stroke, chronic respiratory disease and other conditions. Environmental tobacco smoke and smoking during pregnancy also harm others. Smoking is increasing in many low- and middle-income countries, while steadily, but slowly, decreasing in many high-income countries *(17)*.

Globally, smoking causes about 71% of lung cancer, 42% of chronic respiratory disease and nearly 10% of cardiovascular disease. It is responsible for 12% of male deaths and 6% of female deaths in the world. Tobacco caused an estimated 5.1 million deaths globally in 2004, or almost one in every eight deaths among adults aged 30 years and over (**Table 5**). In India, 11% of deaths in men aged 30–59 years were caused by tobacco smoking.

Death rates for smoking-caused diseases are lower in low-income countries than in middle- and high-income countries (**Figure** 11), reflecting the lower past smoking rates in low-income countries and the higher past smoking rates in high-income countries. Because of the long time lags for development of cancers and chronic respiratory diseases associated with smoking, the impact of smoking-caused diseases on mortality in low- and middle-income countries – and for women in many regions – will continue to rise for at least two decades, even if efforts to reduce smoking are relatively successful.

Alcohol

Alcohol contributes to more than 60 types of disease and injury, although it can also decrease the risk of coronary heart disease, stroke and diabetes. There is wide variation in alcohol consumption across regions. Consumption levels in some Eastern European countries are around 2.5 times higher than the global average of 6.2 litres of pure alcohol per year. With the exception of a few countries, the lowest consumption levels are in Africa and the Eastern Mediterranean.

The net effect of alcohol on cardiovascular disease

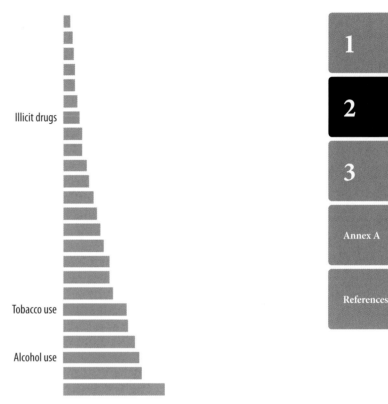

in older people may be protective in regions where alcohol is consumed lightly to moderately in a regular fashion without binge drinking. Ischaemic stroke deaths, for example, would be 11% higher in high-income countries if no one drank alcohol. However, even in high-income countries, although the net impact on cardiovascular disease is beneficial, the overall impact of alcohol on the burden of disease is harmful (**Table 5**).

The regions with the highest proportions of deaths attributed to alcohol were Eastern Europe (more than 1 in every 10 deaths), and Latin America (1 in every 12 deaths). Worldwide, alcohol causes more harm to males (6.0% of deaths, 7.4% of DALYs) than females (1.1% of deaths, 1.4% of DALYs) reflecting differences in drinking habits, both in quantity and pattern of drinking. Besides the direct loss of health due to alcohol addiction, alcohol is responsible for approximately 20% of deaths due to motor vehicle accidents, 30% of deaths due to oesophageal cancer, liver cancer, epilepsy and homicide, and 50% of deaths due to liver cirrhosis.

1
2
3
Annex A
References

Table 5: Deaths and DALYs attributable to alcohol, tobacco and illicit drug use, and to all three risks together, by region, 2004

Risk	World	Low and middle income	High income
Percentage of deaths			
Alcohol use	3.6	4.0	1.6
Illicit drugs	0.4	0.4	0.4
Tobacco use	8.7	7.2	17.9
All three risks	**12.6**	**11.5**	**19.6**
Percentage of DALYs			
Alcohol use	4.4	4.2	6.7
Illicit drugs	0.9	0.8	2.1
Tobacco use	3.7	3.1	10.7
All three risks	**9.0**	**8.1**	**19.2**

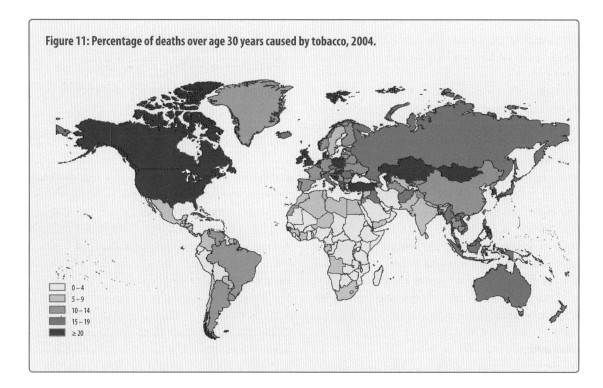

Figure 11: Percentage of deaths over age 30 years caused by tobacco, 2004.

0 – 4
5 – 9
10 – 14
15 – 19
≥ 20

Illicit drug use

Illicit opiate use rose slightly over the period 2000 to 2004, partly due to increased production in Afghanistan, which accounts for 87% of the world's illicit heroin *(18)*. Opiate users are estimated to have risen slightly to around 16 million (11 million using heroin), mostly due to increases in Asia, which contains half of the world's opiate users.

It is difficult to estimate the extent of illegal drug use, and there is considerable uncertainty in the estimated 245 000 deaths attributable to illicit drug use. Dependent users injecting daily for years run the greatest hazard, particularly of HIV/AIDS, overdose, suicide and trauma. Globally, 0.4% of deaths and 0.9% of DALYs were attributed to illicit drug use in 2004. The highest per capita burdens of illicit drug use were in the low- and middle-income countries of the Americas and the Eastern Mediterranean.

2.6 Environmental risks

Unhealthy and unsafe environments cause 1 in 4 child deaths worldwide.

The environment influences the health of people in many ways – through exposures to various physical, chemical and biological risk factors. The five environmental exposures quantified in this report together account for nearly 10% of deaths and disease burden globally (Table 6), and around one quarter of deaths and disease burden in children under 5 years of age.

Unsafe water, sanitation and hygiene

In 2004, 83% of the world's population had some form of improved water supply, while 59% (3.8 billion) had access to basic sanitation facilities *(19)*. Improved drinking-water sources include piped water to the house or yard, public taps or standpipes, boreholes, protected dug wells, protected springs and rainwater collection. Improved sanitation facilities include flush or pour-flush toilets connected to a piped sewer system, septic tanks or pit latrines, and composting toilets.

Inadequate sanitation, hygiene or access to water increase the incidence of diarrhoeal diseases. The highest proportion of deaths and DALYs, as well as the highest absolute numbers, occur in countries with high mortality patterns, such as in Africa and parts of South-East Asia. Most diarrhoeal deaths in the world (88%) is caused by unsafe water, sanitation or hygiene. Overall, more than 99% of these deaths are in developing countries, and around 84% of them occur in children.

Urban outdoor air pollution

Industries, cars and trucks emit complex mixtures of air pollutants, many of which are harmful to health. Of all of these pollutants, fine particulate matter has the greatest effect on human health. Most fine particulate matter comes from fuel combustion, both from mobile sources such as vehicles and from stationary sources such as power plants *(20)*.

Fine particulate matter is associated with a broad spectrum of acute and chronic illness, such as lung cancer and cardiopulmonary disease. Worldwide, it is estimated to cause about 8% of lung cancer deaths,

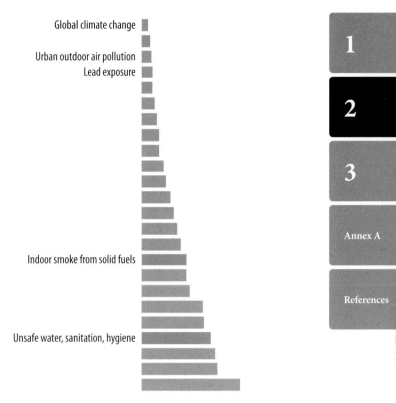

5% of cardiopulmonary deaths and about 3% of respiratory infection deaths. Particulate matter pollution is an environmental health problem that affects people worldwide, but middle-income countries disproportionately experience this burden.

Indoor smoke from solid fuels

More than half the world's population still cooks with wood, dung, coal or agricultural residues on simple stoves or open fires. Especially under conditions of limited ventilation, solid-fuel use leads to high exposures to indoor smoke and large associated health risks, particularly for women and children.

Indoor smoke from solid-fuel use contains a range of potentially harmful substances, from carcinogens to small particulate matter, all of which cause damage to the lungs. Indoor smoke from solid fuel causes about 21% of lower respiratory infection deaths worldwide, 35% of chronic obstructive pulmonary deaths and about 3% of lung cancer deaths. Of these deaths, about 64% occur in low-income countries, especially in South-East Asia and Africa.

Table 6: Deaths and DALYs attributable to five environmental risks, and to all five risks combined by region, 2004.

Risk	World	Low and middle income	High income
Percentage of deaths			
Indoor smoke from solid fuels	3.3	3.9	0.0
Unsafe water, sanitation, hygiene	3.2	3.8	0.1
Urban outdoor air pollution	1.7	1.7	2.1
Global climate change	0.2	0.3	0.0
Lead exposure	0.2	0.3	0.0
All five risks	**9.3**	**10.3**	**2.6**
Percentage of DALYs			
Indoor smoke from solid fuels	2.7	2.9	0.0
Unsafe water, sanitation, hygiene	4.2	4.6	0.3
Urban outdoor air pollution	0.5	0.5	0.8
Global climate change	0.4	0.4	0.0
Lead exposure	0.6	0.6	0.1
All five risks	**8.8**	**9.4**	**1.2**

A further 28% of global deaths caused by indoor smoke from solid fuels occur in China.

Lead exposure

Because of its many uses, lead is present in air, dust, soil and water. Exposure to lead in the womb and during childhood reduces intelligence quotient (IQ), among other behavioural and developmental effects; for adults, it increases blood pressure. Blood lead levels have been steadily declining in industrialized countries following the phasing-out of leaded fuels. However, where leaded petrol is still used, lead can pose a threat, primarily to children in developing countries. Certain populations in industrialized countries are still exposed to high lead levels: mainly from degraded housing. Overall, 98% of adults and 99% of children affected by exposure to lead live in low- and middle-income countries.

Climate change

Average global temperatures are likely to rise by 1.1–6.4 °C between 1990 and 2100 *(21)*. Physical, ecological and social factors will have a complex effect on climate change. Because of this complexity, current estimates of the attributable and avoidable impacts of climate change are based on models with considerable uncertainty.

Potential risks to health include deaths from thermal extremes and weather disasters, vector-borne diseases, a higher incidence of food-related and waterborne infections, photochemical air pollutants and conflict over depleted natural resources. Climate change will have the greatest effect on health in societies with scarce resources, little technology and frail infrastructure. Only some of the many potential effects were fully quantifiable; for example, the effects of more frequent and extreme storms were excluded. Climate change was estimated to be already responsible for 3% of diarrhoea, 3% of malaria and 3.8% of dengue fever deaths worldwide in 2004. Total attributable mortality was about 0.2% of deaths in 2004; of these, 85% were child deaths. In addition, increased temperatures hastened as many as 12 000 additional deaths; however these deaths were not included in the totals because the years of life lost by these individuals were uncertain, and possibly brief.

2.7   Occupational and other risks

Occupational noise exposure causes about 16% of adult-onset hearing loss.
Unsafe health-care injections cause more deaths in low- and middle-income countries than colon and rectum cancer.

People face numerous hazards at work, which may result in injuries, cancer, hearing loss, and respiratory, musculoskeletal, cardiovascular, reproductive, neurological, skin and mental disorders. This report evaluates only selected risk factors because of the lack of global data, but these occupational risks alone account for 1.7% of DALYs lost worldwide. In addition, there is increasing evidence from industrialized countries to link coronary heart disease and depression with work-related stress *(3, 22)*.

Occupational injuries
Overall, more than 350 000 workers lose their lives each year due to unintentional occupational injuries. More than 90% of this injury burden is borne by men and more than half of the global burden occurs among men working in the WHO South-East Asia and Western Pacific regions. In men aged 15–59 years, 8% of the total burden of unintentional injury is attributable to work-related injuries in high-income countries, and 18% in low- and middle-income countries.

Occupational carcinogens
At least 150 chemical and biological agents are known or probable causes of cancer. Many of these are found in the workplace, even though occupational cancers are almost entirely preventable through eliminating exposure, substituting safer materials, enclosing processes and ventilation. Worldwide, these occupational exposures account for an estimated 8% of lung cancer, which is the most frequent form of occupational cancer.

Occupational airborne particulates
Workplace exposure to microscopic airborne particles can cause lung cancer, chronic obstructive pulmonary disease, silicosis, asbestosis and pneumoconiosis. These diseases take a long time to develop, so,

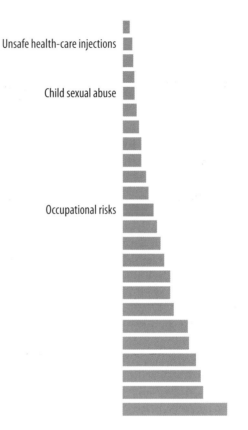

even in countries where the risk has been recognized and controlled, the rate of decline in disease burden has been slow. In developing countries, trends are mostly unknown, but the problem is substantial. Occupational exposure to airborne particulates is estimated to cause 12% of deaths due to chronic obstructive pulmonary disease. Additionally, an estimated 29 000 deaths are due to silicosis, asbestosis and pneumoconiosis caused by silica, asbestos and coal dust exposure.

Ergonomic stressors
Low back pain can be caused by lifting and carrying heavy loads, demanding physical work, frequent bending, twisting and awkward postures. Such pain is rarely life-threatening, but can limit work and social activities. An estimated 37% of back pain is attributable to occupational risk factors. Although not a cause of premature mortality, low back pain causes considerable morbidity and is a major cause of work absences, resulting in economic loss.

Occupational noise

Excess noise is one of the most common occupational hazards, particularly for mining, manufacturing and construction workers, especially in developing countries. Its most serious effect is irreversible hearing impairment, which is completely preventable. Most exposure can be minimized by engineering controls to reduce noise at its source. About 16% of adult-onset hearing loss worldwide is attributable to occupational noise exposure. According to the WHO definition of hearing loss (23), this corresponds to 4.5 million DALYs for moderate or greater levels of hearing loss. Mild hearing loss was not included in this estimate.

Unsafe health-care injections

The complexity of modern health care inevitably brings risks as well as benefits. Patient safety is a serious global public health issue. Estimates show that, in developed countries, as many as 1 patient in 10 is harmed while receiving hospital care.

The probability of patients being harmed in hospitals is higher in developing countries than in industrialized nations. The risk of health-care associated infection in some developing countries is up to 20 times higher than in developed countries. Mortality rates associated with major surgery are also unacceptably high in many developing countries (24). The situation in developing countries may also be made worse because of the use of counterfeit and substandard drugs, and inappropriate or poor equipment and infrastructure.

Injections are overused in many countries, and unsafe injections cause many infections: in particular hepatitis B and C, and HIV. Unsafe injections result mainly from the reuse of injection equipment without adequately sterilizing it. Unsafe injections account for an estimated 30% of hepatitis B infections, 24% of hepatitis C infections, 27% of liver cancer, 24% of liver cirrhosis deaths and 1.3% of HIV deaths worldwide. An estimated 417 000 people died as a result of disease transmitted by unsafe injections in 2004.

Child sex abuse

Child sex abuse increases the risk of a range of mental disorders in adult life, including depression, anxiety disorders, drug or alcohol abuse, and suicide. The percentage of adults who have been sexually abused during childhood ranged from around 4% of men in high-income countries to more than 40% of women in parts of Africa and Asia. About one third of post-traumatic stress disorder cases in women and one fifth in men are attributable to child sex abuse (25). Between 5 and 8% of alcohol and drug use disorders are attributable to child sex abuse. Much of the burden of child sex abuse is disabling rather than fatal, and occurs in the young. Applying these fractions to DALY estimates for 2004 resulted in 0.6% of the global burden of disease being attributable to child sex abuse.

Other health risks

Many thousands of other threats to health exist within and outside the categories considered in this report. They include risk factors for tuberculosis and malaria (together responsible for 4.5% of the global disease burden), family environment risk factors for mental disorders, risk factors for injuries, and a complex range of dietary risks. Some important risks associated with exposure to infectious disease agents or with antimicrobial resistance are also not included. Genetics play a substantial role, although this report has not attempted to quantify the attributable burden of disease from genetic causes. In general, this report's approach and methodology can be applied more widely; as a result, the potential for prevention of other risks to health can be brought to the attention of health policy-makers.

More than 90% of road deaths occur in low- and middle-income countries, where the death rates (20 and 22 per 100 000 population, respectively) are almost double those for high-income countries. Because many deaths occur in young adults, the loss of potential healthy life is great (26).

Crashes are largely preventable using engineering measures – such as traffic management – vehicle design and equipment such as helmets and seat belts, and road-user measures such as speed limits (27). When used correctly, seat belts reduce the risk of death in a crash by 61%. In Thailand, a motorcycle helmet law cut deaths by 56%, and it has been estimated that lowering average speeds by 5 km per hour would cut deaths by 25% in Western Europe. If countries with high rates of road injury were able to reduce road death rates to the best levels achieved in their regions, global road fatalities would fall by 44%.

Intentional injuries caused 1.6 million deaths in 2004: 51% of these by suicide, 37% by violence between individuals, and 11% in wars and civil conflict. Interpersonal violence was the second leading cause of death in 2004 among men aged 15–44 years, after road traffic accidents. There is a close relationship between violence and poverty; countries with lower per capita income have higher homicide rates, but rates were substantially higher in the low- and middle-income countries of Africa and the Americas than in other regions. Other risk factors for interpersonal violence include alcohol and availability of weapons, particularly firearms.

Collective violence, including war, caused an estimated 184 000 deaths in 2004 – more than half of these in the WHO Eastern Mediterranean Region, and half of the remainder in Africa (2). Risk factors for collective violence include the wide availability of small arms, political and socioeconomic inequalities, and abuse of human rights.

1

2

3

Annex A

References

3 Joint effects of risk factors

3.1 Joint contribution of risk factors to specific diseases

Many diseases are caused by more than one risk factor, and thus may be prevented by reducing any of the risk factors responsible for them. As a result, the sum of the mortality or burden of disease attributable to each of the risk factors separately is often more than the combined mortality and burden of disease attributable to the groups of these risk factors.

For example, of all infectious and parasitic child deaths (including those caused by acute lower respiratory infections), 34% can be attributed to underweight; 26% to unsafe water, hygiene and sanitation; and 15% to smoke from indoor use of solid fuels. The joint effect of all three of these risk factors is, however, 46%. Similarly, 45% of cardiovascular deaths among those older than 30 years can be attributed to raised blood pressure, 16% to raised cholesterol and 13% to raised blood glucose, yet the estimated combined effect of these three risks is about 48% of cardiovascular diseases.

Risks for child health

In 2004, 10.4 million children under 5 years of age died: 45% in the WHO African Region and 30% in the South-East Asia Region. The leading causes of death among children under 5 years of age are acute respiratory infections and diarrhoeal diseases, which are also the leading overall causes of loss of healthy life years. Child underweight is the leading individual risk for child deaths and loss of healthy life years, causing 21% of deaths and DALYs. Child underweight, together with micronutrient deficiencies and suboptimal breastfeeding, accounted for 35% of child deaths and 32% of loss of healthy life years worldwide. Unsafe water, sanitation and hygiene, together with indoor smoke from solid fuels, cause 23% of child deaths. These environmental risks, together with the nutritional risks and suboptimal breastfeeding, cause 39% of child deaths worldwide.

Risks for cardiovascular disease

The two leading causes of death are cardiovascular – ischaemic heart disease and cerebrovascular disease;

cardiovascular diseases account for nearly 30% of deaths worldwide. Eight risk factors – alcohol use, tobacco use, high blood pressure, high body mass index, high cholesterol, high blood glucose, low fruit and vegetable intake, and physical inactivity – account for 61% of loss of healthy life years from cardiovascular diseases and 61% of cardiovascular deaths. The same risk factors together account for over three quarters of deaths from ischaemic and hypertensive heart disease.

Cardiovascular deaths occur at older ages in high-income countries than in low- and middle-income countries. DALYs account for this difference by giving a higher weight to deaths at younger ages. Among adults over 30 years of age, the rate of DALYs attributed to the eight cardiovascular risk factors is more than twice as high in middle-income European countries than in high-income countries or in the Western Pacific Region, where rates are lowest. In all regions, the leading cause of cardiovascular death is high blood pressure, which causes between 37% of cardiovascular deaths in the South-East Asia Region to 54% of cardiovascular deaths in middle-income European countries. The eight cardiovascular risk factors cause the largest proportion of cardiovascular deaths in middle-income European countries (72%) and the smallest proportion in African countries (51%).

Risks for cancer

Cancer rates are increased by many of the risks considered in this report, and some leading cancers could be substantially reduced by lowering exposure to these risks. Worldwide, 71% of lung cancer deaths are caused by tobacco use (lung cancer is the leading cause of cancer death globally). The combined effects of tobacco use, low fruit and vegetable intake, urban air pollution, and indoor smoke from household use of solid fuels cause 76% of lung cancer deaths. All deaths and unhealthy life years from cervical cancer are caused by human papillomavirus infection from unsafe sex. Nine leading environmental and behavioural risks – high body mass index, low fruit and vegetable intake, physical inactivity, tobacco use, alcohol use, unsafe sex, urban and indoor air pollution, and unsafe health-care injections – are responsible for 35% of cancer deaths.

Cancers are also caused by infections. Worldwide,

63% of stomach cancer deaths are caused by infection with *Helicobacter pylori*, 73% of liver cancer deaths are caused by infection with viral hepatitis or liver flukes, and 100% of cervical cancer deaths are caused by infection with human papillomavirus. The combined effects of seven infectious agents – blood and liver flukes, human papillomavirus, hepatitis B and C, herpesvirus and *H. pylori* – cause 18% of cancer deaths. Together with the nine environmental and behavioural causes of cancer, these infections explain 45% of cancer deaths worldwide. For specific cancer sites, the proportion is higher: more than three quarters of deaths from mouth and oropharynx cancer, liver cancer, lung cancer and cervical cancer can be explained by infections, and environmental and behavioural exposures.

3.2 Potential health gains from reducing multiple risk factors

Reducing or eliminating the risks described in this report could reduce by three quarters or more the deaths and DALYs caused by leading diseases such as ischaemic heart disease, diabetes, diarrhoea and HIV/AIDS (**Figure 12**). Nearly one half (44%) of deaths in the world in the year 2004 could be attributed to the 24 risk factors analysed in this report, when joint effects were taken into account (**Table 7**). One third (33%) of global deaths could be attributed to the leading 10 risk factors (defined by total attributable burden), and more than one quarter to the leading five risk factors (25%). The leading 10 risk factors were responsible for one quarter of the total loss of healthy years of life globally.

The risks considered in this report explain a larger proportion of loss of healthy years of life in Africa and low- and middle-income European countries (40% and 45%) than in other regions, where these risk factors cause about one third of the loss of healthy years of life. This is because of the importance of cardiovascular risk factors, including alcohol, in Europe, and child risks, as well as risks for HIV/AIDS, in Africa.

Had these 24 risks not existed, life expectancy would have been on average almost a decade longer in 2004 for the entire global population (**Figure 13**). Low and middle income countries have much more to gain than the richest countries: for example, life

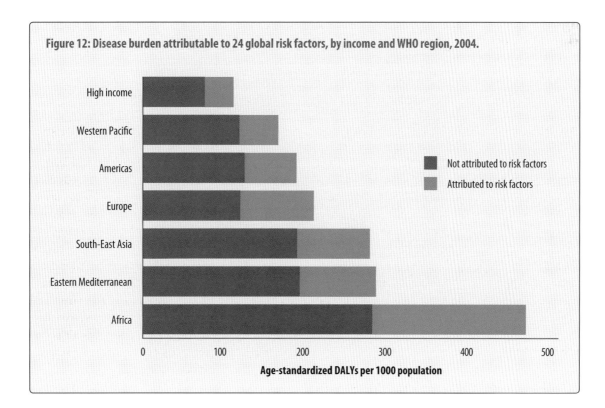

Figure 12: Disease burden attributable to 24 global risk factors, by income and WHO region, 2004.

Legend:
- Not attributed to risk factors
- Attributed to risk factors

Age-standardized DALYs per 1000 population

Table 7: Percentage of total disease burden due to 5 and 10 leading risks and all 24 risks in this report, world, 2004

	5 leading risks	10 leading risks	24 risks
Attributable deaths (%)	25	33	44
Attributable DALYs (%)	20	25	35
Attributable life expectancy loss (years)	4.9	6.8	9.3

Table 8: Percentage of total disease burden due to 10 leading risks, by region and income group, 2004

	Region						
	High income	Africa	Americas	Eastern Mediter-ranean	Europe	South-East Asia	Western Pacific
Attributable deaths (%)	28	40	34	31	49	29	29
Attributable DALYs (%)	21	34	24	21	34	22	19
Attributable life expectancy loss (years)	3.3	11.3	5.6	6.4	8.8	5.8	4.0

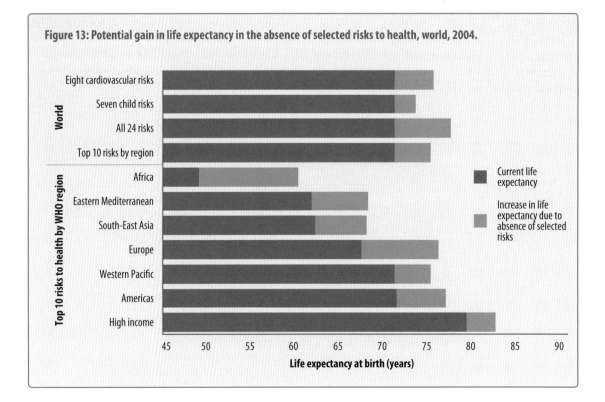

Figure 13: Potential gain in life expectancy in the absence of selected risks to health, world, 2004.

expectancy would have grown by nearly 13 years in the African Region, but by less than 6 years in the high-income countries. The five leading risks alone shortened life expectancy by about 9 years in Africa in 2004.

3.3   Conclusions

It is clear that the world faces some large, widespread and certain risks to health. The five leading risk factors identified in this report are responsible for one quarter of all deaths in the world; all 24 risk factors are responsible for almost one half of all deaths. Although some of these major risk factors (e.g. tobacco use or overweight and obesity) are usually associated with high-income countries, in fact, more than three quarters of the total global burden of diseases they cause already occurs in low- and middle-income countries. Health risks are in transition – and health has become globalized – as patterns of consumption change markedly around the world and populations contain higher proportions of older people, as a result of successes against infectious diseases and decreasing fertility levels.

Developing countries increasingly face a double burden from the risks for communicable diseases and maternal and child outcomes that traditionally affect the poor combined with the risks for noncommunicable conditions. The poorest countries still face a high and concentrated burden from poverty, undernutrition, unsafe sex, unsafe water and sanitation, iron deficiency and indoor smoke from solid fuels. At the same time, dietary risk factors for high blood pressure, cholesterol and obesity, coupled with insufficient physical activity, are responsible for an increasing proportion of the total disease burden. Had the risks considered in this report not existed, life expectancy would have been on average almost a decade longer in 2004 for the entire global population, with greater increases in the low-income countries than in the high-income countries.

The results from the report provide powerful input for policy actions when combined with information about interventions, their costs and their efficacy. Although risk exposure estimates are based on less-than-perfect data, they are often conservative because, as health improves, gains can multiply. For example, reducing the burden of disease in the poor may raise income levels, which, in turn, will further help to reduce health inequalities. Many cost-effective interventions are also known, and prevention strategies can be transferred between similar countries. Much of the necessary scientific and economic information, evidence and research is already available for guiding policy decisions that could significantly improve global health.

Annex A: Data and methods

For *The world health report 2002*, WHO developed a new framework for quantifying deaths and burden of disease caused by risk factors, with an emphasis on improving the comparability of the estimates *(1)*. Different risk factors have very different epidemiological traditions, particularly with regard to defining "hazardous" exposure, the strength of evidence on causality, and the availability of epidemiological research on exposure and outcomes. Moreover, classical risk factor research has treated exposures as dichotomous, with individuals either exposed or not exposed, and with exposure defined according to a threshold value that is often arbitrary. Recent evidence for such continuous exposures as cholesterol, blood pressure and body mass index suggests that such arbitrarily defined thresholds are inappropriate because hazard functions for these risks change continuously across the entire range of measured exposure levels, with no obvious threshold *(e.g., 28)*.

The risk factor burden was calculated for *The world health report 2002* as the reduction in disease burden that would be expected under the risk factor exposure scenario that minimizes risk *(29, 30)*. Fractions of disease burden attributable to a risk factor were calculated based on a comparison of disease burden observed under the current distribution of exposure by age, sex and region, with that expected if a counterfactual distribution of exposure had applied. To improve comparability across risk factors, a counterfactual distribution was defined for each risk factor as the population distribution of exposure that would lead to the lowest levels of disease burden. This counterfactual exposure is assumed to have applied in the reference year and in all previous years.

For this update of global estimates of mortality and burden of disease attributable to 24 global risk factors, the methods developed for *The world health report 2002* were applied, with updated inputs on exposure distributions for 2004 and, in some cases, updated estimates of the magnitude of the hazards associated with specific risk exposures. These revisions are documented below. Two new risk factors were included for the first time in this update: suboptimal breastfeeding and higher-than-optimal blood glucose. Regional-level estimates of mortality

and DALYs for specific diseases and injuries for 2004 were from a recent WHO update of global burden of disease estimates *(2)*. For some risk factors – including fruit and vegetable intake, occupation risk factors, child sexual abuse and unsafe health-care injections – revised estimates of exposure distributions were not available, and disease- and injury-specific population attributable fractions (PAFs) calculated for the year 2000 were assumed also to apply in 2004.

A1.1 Estimating population attributable fractions

To calculate the difference in population health under the counterfactual scenario, the PAF is first calculated. PAF is defined as:

$$PAF = \frac{\int\limits_{x=0}^{m} RR(x)P(x)dx - \int\limits_{x=0}^{m} RR(x)P'(x)dx}{\int\limits_{x=0}^{m} RR(x)P(x)dx} \qquad (1)$$

where $RR(x)$ = relative risk at each exposure level, $P(x)$ = proportion of population at each exposure level, $P'(x)$ = counterfactual proportion of population at each exposure level, and m = maximum exposure level *(31)*.

For risk factors where the exposure is dichotomous (exposed, not exposed), and the counterfactual scenario is no exposure, equation 1 reduces to equation 2:

$$PAF = P \cdot (RR - 1)/[P \cdot (RR - 1) + 1] \qquad (2)$$

where P = prevalence of exposure, and RR = relative risk for exposed versus non-exposed.

Once the fraction of a disease (or injury) that is attributed to a risk factor has been established, the attributable mortality or burden is simply the product of the total death or DALY estimates for the disease and the attributable fraction. For most diseases, the same attributable fraction is applied to fatal (YLL) and non-fatal (YLD) burden estimates.

Choice of counterfactual

Analysis using counterfactual exposure distributions requires comparing the current distributions of exposure to risk factors with some alternative distribution. We used the theoretical minimum risk distribution – that is, the distribution of exposure that would yield the lowest population risk – in analyses for this report *(29)*. The theoretical minimum exposure distribution may be zero in some cases because zero exposure reflects minimum risk (e.g. no smoking). For some risk factors, zero exposure is an inappropriate choice because these are physiologically impossible (e.g. body mass index and cholesterol). For these risk factors, the lowest levels observed in specific populations and epidemiological studies were used in choosing the theoretical minimum.

In the case of tobacco, for example, the counterfactual exposure distribution that gives minimum-risk would be that 100% of the population were life-long non-smokers; whereas, for overweight and obesity, it would be a narrow distribution of body mass index centred around an optimal level (e.g. mean 21 (standard deviation 1) kg/m²), and so on. The theoretical minimum risk exposure distributions for the risk factors quantified here are listed in Table A1.

Joint effects of risk factors

We also calculated the fraction of mortality attributed to the combined effects of these risk factors. Among those people exposed to multiple risk factors, disease-specific deaths may be caused by the simultaneous effects of multiple exposures, and hence can be prevented by reducing exposure to any of the risks. For example, some deaths from ischaemic heart disease may be prevented by reducing blood pressure or by reducing cholesterol. As a result of multicausality, the PAFs for multiple risk factors cannot be combined by simple addition *(32)*. The combined (joint) PAF that avoids double counting the overlap of multiple risk factors is given by equation 3 *(33)*:

$$PAF = 1 - \prod_{i=1}^{n}(1 - PAF_i) \qquad (3)$$

where PAF_i = PAF for individual risk factor i, and n = total number of risk factors that affect the same disease outcome.

Equation 3 is based on three specific assumptions about the correlation of the exposures to the multiple risks and the interactions of their causal effects *(33)*. Firstly, it assumes that the exposure to the risk factors is uncorrelated within a given country. Secondly, it assumes that the level of exposure to one risk factor does not affect the proportional increase in risk caused by another (i.e. no effect modification). Thirdly, it assumes that the effect of one risk factor does not act through another (i.e. no mediated effects). We accounted for instances where these assumptions are violated based on methods published elsewhere *(9, 33)*. For example, we accounted for the increased risk of ischaemic heart disease caused by physical inactivity that acts through increased blood pressure. In previous analyses, neither high blood glucose nor infectious causes of cancer (see page 40) were considered as independent risk factors. It is likely that some proportion of the burden of high body mass index acts through high blood glucose. In analysis of the Framingham Offspring Study cohort, Wilson et al. found that approximately two thirds of the effect of body mass index is mediated through cholesterol, blood pressure and blood glucose; we therefore reduced the burden of body mass index by two thirds before calculating the joint effect of the risk factors *(34)*. We assumed that infectious causes of cancer act independently of the behavioural and environmental causes of cancer considered in this report, with the exception of the risk factors that increase burden by infection, such as the effect of unsafe injections on liver cancer.

A1.2 Risk factors

This section describes the methods used for each of the 24 risk factors included in this report. A summary of the exposure variable, counterfactual exposure levels, disease outcomes, and sources of exposure and hazard estimates is provided in Table A1, and estimated exposure prevalences in Table A2. Tables A3 and A4 provide a summary of the attributable mortality and DALYs for all 24 risk factors for the world, males, females and populations, grouped by country average income per capita.

Childhood and maternal underweight

The prevalence of child underweight was based on analysis of 388 nationally representative studies for

139 countries from the WHO Global Database on Child Growth and Malnutrition.[1] These were used to estimate prevalence of child underweight (for z-score categories of body mass index <-3, -3 to <-2, -2 to <-1) for each country in the world according to the new WHO Child Growth Standards (35-38). The prevalences of maternal underweight (body mass index < 20 kg/m²) were derived from country-level estimates of means and standard deviations for body mass index from the WHO *Surveillance of chronic disease risk factors* report (SuRF report 2) (39).

Disease-specific relative risks for mortality associated with childhood underweight were estimated by Black et al. (9) using eight data sets from low-income countries (Bangladesh, Ghana, Guinea-Bissau, India, Nepal, the Philippines, Pakistan and Senegal). The estimated risks were then adjusted for confounding due to socioeconomic factors that affect mortality through other pathways, such as non-nutritional determinants of infection or access to better clinical care. The same relative risks as for mortality were used for diarrhoea, pneumonia and malaria morbidity.

The CRA 2000 study (40) also estimated the proportion of neonatal mortality and morbidity due to low birth weight that was attributable to maternal underweight. Black et al. (9) estimated the attributable fractions for birth asphyxia/trauma and neonatal infections attributable to intrauterine growth restriction (IUGR) in babies born at term (i.e. who have completed 37 weeks of gestation). Data from five community-sampled prospective birth cohorts in developing countries were analysed to estimate relative risks of neonatal death due to birth asphyxia and infections (sepsis, pneumonia and diarrhoea). The results presented here include the attributable mortality and burden for neonatal outcomes associated with IUGR due to maternal underweight, and assuming that IUGR deaths were only 0.4% of total neonatal deaths (2).

Iron deficiency

Anaemia prevalence distributions were updated for 2004 using data collected for the Vitamin and Mineral Nutrition Information System[2] by the WHO Department of Nutrition for Health and Development for preschool-aged children, pregnant women and non-pregnant women. These estimates were based on the most recent national and subnational surveys measuring blood haemoglobin concentration carried out in the years 1993–2005 (11). According to these estimates, 42% of pregnant women and 47% of preschool children worldwide have anaemia. Following previous global burden of disease estimates, the 2004 GBD report assumed that 60% of anaemia was due to iron deficiency in non-malaria areas and 50% in malaria areas (2).

Deaths and DALYs estimated for the global burden of disease cause category "iron-deficiency anaemia" were attributed 100% to iron deficiency. These DALYs include the direct impact of anaemia on functioning at all ages in both sexes, and the impact on cognitive functioning in children (2). In addition, anaemia in pregnancy is considered a risk factor for maternal mortality. The attributable mortality and disease burden for maternal causes was estimated using the methods and assumptions of Stoltzfus et al. (41). Following Black et al., we did not consider the effect of iron deficiency on perinatal mortality (9). Country-specific distributions for anaemia in 2004, and for the theoretical minimum counterfactual distributions, were updated using anaemia prevalence estimates for pregnant women for 2004 (11).

Vitamin A deficiency

Exposure data and hazard estimates were updated using recently published updates for country and regional prevalence of vitamin A deficiency in children and new estimates of the relative risks for cause-specific mortality (9). Exposures were estimated based on the percentage of children under 5 years of age living in areas classified as vitamin A deficient, based on population survey data for low plasma or tissue retinol levels and xerophthalmia, together with information on coverage of vitamin A supplementation programmes.

Blindness from corneal scarring directly due to xerophthalmia is 100% attributed to vitamin A deficiency. The relative risks for mortality due to diarrhoea and measles as a result of vitamin A deficiency

---

[1] http://www.who.int/nutgrowthdb/
[2] http://www.who.int/vmnis

were derived from a meta-analysis of nine randomized placebo-controlled trials in children aged 6–59 months showing risk reduction with supplementation *(42)*. The findings from three trials of vitamin A supplementation of newborns were used to estimate relative risks for mortality from neonatal infections and from prematurity *(9)*. These trials, which were conducted in Bangladesh, India and Indonesia, showed reductions in mortality during infancy ranging from 15% to 64%. However, three other trials conducted in Guinea-Bissau, Nepal and Zimbabwe have shown no effect of this intervention on infant mortality.

Pooled results from trials did not show a consistent association of vitamin A deficiency with malaria mortality or morbidity, or an increased risk of maternal mortality *(9)*. These disease endpoints were therefore not included in the analysis for vitamin A deficiency.

Zinc deficiency

Exposure data and hazard estimates were updated using recently published estimates of country and regional prevalence of zinc deficiency in children under 5 years of age, and new estimates of the relative risks for mortality and morbidity due to diarrhoeal diseases, lower respiratory tract infections and malaria *(9)*. The child population's risk of zinc deficiency was estimated for the 178 countries for which food availability information was available from the Food and Agriculture Organization of the United Nations. The latest prevalence of stunting for 131 countries was obtained from the WHO Global Database on Child Growth and Malnutrition *(35-38)*. Data from other sources were used to classify 35 additional countries by prevalence of stunting. The total child population of each country was classified as zinc deficient or not zinc deficient based on the combination of the prevalence of stunting and adequacy of zinc in the food supply. Relative risks for diarrhoea, pneumonia and malaria incidence in children due to zinc deficiency were estimated from a meta-analysis of placebo-controlled trials *(9)*.

Suboptimal breastfeeding

We based our analysis on the methods of Black et al., who recently published an analysis of the global burden of suboptimal breastfeeding *(9)*. Black et al.

provide data for breastfeeding levels for 30 developing countries and 12 regions, mainly covering the developing world. Data were limited for developed countries; therefore, prevalence estimates from the United States of America (USA) and Australia were used *(43, 44)*. The breastfeeding prevalence for the USA was applied to all high-income countries that were not covered by Black et al. and were not located in the WHO Western Pacific Region. Breastfeeding prevalence from Australia was applied to all Western Pacific countries not covered by Black et al. In this analysis, relative risks for diarrhoeal diseases, lower respiratory tract infections and infectious perinatal conditions were calculated for children aged under 24 months. Relative risks were calculated for these conditions across four exposure categories (exclusive, predominant, partial and non-breastfeeding) in the 0–5 months age group and two (any and non-breastfeeding) in the 6–23 month age group. Relative risks and prevalence data for perinatal infections were estimated only for the 0–1 month age group for all countries. Optimal breastfeeding is defined as exclusive breastfeeding for the first 6 months of life and continued breastfeeding through the second year of life *(9)*.

High blood pressure

WHO's *SuRF report 2* presents estimates of mean population blood pressure for 192 Member States, as well as standard deviations *(39)*. Estimates were made using available survey data standardized for age groups and reporting year with regression analysis. Estimates for 2004 were used in this analysis. Relative risks were from the Prospective Studies Collaboration: a meta-analysis of 61 studies *(45)*. Following the CRA 2000 study, we used a counterfactual population systolic blood pressure distribution with a mean of 115 mmHg and a standard deviation of 6 mmHg.

High cholesterol

Mean total serum cholesterol and standard deviation for 2004 were from WHO's *SuRF report 2 (39)*. Relative risks were from the prospective studies collaboration: a meta-analysis of 61 studies *(28)*. We used a counterfactual population serum cholesterol distribution with a mean of 3.8 mmol/l and a standard deviation of 0.5 mmol/l.

High body mass index

Mean body mass index and standard deviation for 2004 were from WHO's *SuRF report 2 (39)*. Relative risks for colon, uterine and post-menopausal breast cancer were from a recent meta-analysis of 221 data sets *(46)*. All other relative risks were from the Asia Pacific Cohort Studies collaboration: a meta-analysis of 33 cohorts *(47, 48)*. We used a counterfactual population body mass index distribution with a mean of 21 kg/m^2 and a standard deviation of 1 kg/m^2.

Low fruit and vegetable intake

We used the estimated regional mean and standard deviation of fruit and vegetable consumption for 2000 from Lock et al. *(49)*. Following Danaei et al. *(50)*, we used relative risks from several recent meta-analyses. Relative risks for ischaemic heart disease were from Dauchet et al. *(51)*, for ischaemic stroke from Dauchet et al. *(52)*, for oesophageal cancer from Boeing et al. *(53)*, and for lung, stomach, colon and rectum cancers from Lock et al. *(49)*. We also used the theoretical minimum risk distribution of fruit and vegetable consumption hypothesized by Lock et al. (fruit and vegetable consumption: mean 600 g/day, standard deviation 50 g/day) as the counterfactual.

Physical inactivity

The CRA 2000 study categorized physical activity into three levels – inactive, insufficiently active and sufficiently active – with the counterfactual exposure distribution being 100% sufficiently active *(54)*. Recent CRA studies have treated physical inactivity as a four-level categorical variable by subdividing the "sufficiently active" exposure group into those "meeting current recommendations" and "highly active" *(50, 55)*. Although physical activity levels equivalent to 2.5 hours per week of moderate-intensity activity or 1 hour per week of vigorous activity – approximately equivalent to 600 MET (metabolic equivalent; that is, energy expenditure measured in units of resting energy expenditure) minutes per week – are considered an important target for population health benefits, the protective effects are expected to continue at higher levels. For this update, four exposure categories were used: dividing the "sufficiently active" exposure group into "moderately active" and

"highly active". The threshold for "highly active" was physical activity levels equivalent to at least 1 hour per week of vigorous activity and a total energy expenditure of 1600 MET minutes per week. The theoretical minimum risk exposure distribution was chosen as the whole population being in the "highly active" category to increase consistency of the counterfactual exposure distribution with those for other risk factors and with the definition of theoretical minimum risk *(50, 55)*.

For this update, we used regional prevalence distributions estimated for the CRA 2000 study, with the "sufficiently active" prevalence split into "moderately" and "highly" active using data from the Global Physical Activity Questionnaire (GPAQ), implemented in 28 countries using the WHO Stepwise approach to chronic disease risk factor surveillance (STEPS) approach *(56)*. Age-specific and sex-specific fractions for the "highly active" as a proportion of the "sufficiently active" were estimated for the CRA 2000 subregions based on the subregional average income per capita in 2004, using the GPAQ data for 28 mainly low- and middle-income countries, together with recent data for the USA *(50)* to fit age-specific and sex-specific linear regressions on the log of gross national income per capita. The regression slopes were quite consistent across age and sex groups. The resulting prevalence distributions are summarized in Table A.2.

Relative risks consistent with the four-category exposure have been developed by Begg et al. *(55)* and Danaei et al. *(50)*; we used the latter estimates because they were based on the 2000 CRA analysis *(54)*, modified to correspond to the new referent category of "highly active". The revised estimates for mortality and DALYs attributable to physical inactivity for 2004 are higher than the 2000 estimates, with most of the increase being due to mortality among the "inactive" and "insufficiently active" groups assessed against the new referent category. Improved estimates of population distributions of physical activity from the GPAQ and other new survey data sources may result in future revisions to these estimates.

High blood glucose

In addition to deaths and burden of disease directly assigned to diabetes under the rules of the

International Classification of Diseases, mortality from cardiovascular diseases is also higher in people with diabetes, and cardiovascular mortality risk increases continuously with blood glucose concentration, from levels well below the threshold levels used in the definition of diabetes (8). Mortality and disease burden attributable to higher-than-optimal blood glucose are included in this report, using the methods and regional blood glucose concentration estimates developed by Danaei et al. (8). Regional exposure distributions were estimated using measurements of fasting plasma glucose (FPG) concentration from 65 population studies in 52 countries. The theoretical minimum (counterfactual) distribution for FPG was based on the lowest observed distribution in younger adults with mean of 4.9 mmol/l and standard deviation of 0.3 mmol/l. In addition to diabetes mellitus with PAF of 100%, PAFs were estimated for ischaemic heart disease and cerebrovascular disease using relative risks derived from the Asia Pacific Cohort Study meta-analysis of 13 cohorts with 200 000 participants from the WHO regions of South-East Asia and the Western Pacific (57).

Unsafe sex

All sexually transmitted diseases are attributed to unsafe sex. The PAFs for HIV/AIDS and hepatitis B and C due to unsafe sex were derived as described by Slaymaker et al. (58). PAFs were updated for 2004 using country and regional estimates of transmission mode proportions for unsafe sex from UNAIDS monitoring reports and other publications (59-64). All cervical cancer is attributed to sexual transmission of human papillomavirus (65).

Lack of contraception

Non-use and use of ineffective methods of contraception increases the risk of maternal morbidity and mortality associated with unwanted and mistimed births and with unsafe abortion. We used the methods developed by Collumbien et al. for the CRA 2000 study (66). Regional exposure data were updated using most recent country-level data on annual average time trends in the prevalence of use of modern and traditional contraceptive methods, and prevalence of non-use of contraception for the period 1997–2007 (67). Relative risks for unsafe abortion and for maternal conditions – such as

maternal haemorrhage, maternal sepsis, hypertensive disorders of pregnancy, obstructed labour and other maternal conditions – were from the CRA 2000 study (66).

Smoking and oral tobacco use

Smoking intensity, average age at initiation and average duration vary considerably from setting to setting and by sex. Using the reported prevalence of smoking in a population would thus bias the calculation of the attributable burden. Therefore, following previous CRA analyses, we used the method of Peto et al., who proposed that current incidence of lung cancer can be used as an indicator of past exposure to tobacco smoke (68). We calculated a "smoking impact ratio" by comparing lung cancer mortality rates in each population with lung cancer mortality rates among non-smokers and smokers observed in the American Cancer Society study: a large long-term follow-up study in the United States (69). Chewing tobacco is an important cause of oral and oesophageal cancers in South Asia. For Bangladesh, India and Pakistan, we estimated oral tobacco use using reported tobacco use in the India World Health Survey (70). Because chewing tobacco is rare in other parts of the world, we did not consider its effects beyond South Asia.

Relative risks of smoking from the American Cancer Society study have recently been updated, and age-specific relative risks were modelled by Danaei et al. (50). We used the relative risks for cancers (lung, upper aerodigestive tract, stomach, cancer, pancreas, cervix uteri, bladder, leukaemia, colon and rectum), selected cardiovascular causes of death, chronic obstructive pulmonary disease and other respiratory causes used by Danaei et al., but originally reported elsewhere (69, 71, 72). Danaie et al. only considered the effect of smoking on hypertensive heart disease in their sensitivity analysis, although the effect is consistently observed (72); because of the importance of hypertensive heart disease worldwide, we included this effect in our primary analysis. Relative risks for tuberculosis and for the effect of chewing tobacco were not available from the American Cancer Society cohort; instead, we used relative risks for tuberculosis from Lin et al. (73), and from Rao et al. for the effect of chewing tobacco on upper aerodigestive tract cancers (74).

We compared current tobacco use with an ideal scenario of no tobacco use.

Alcohol

Estimates for direct deaths and DALYs due to alcohol dependence and harmful use (alcohol use disorders) in 2004 were revised based on a new review of population studies, published data on alcohol production, trade and sales, and health state valuations collected in the WHO Multi-Country Survey Study *(75)*.

For other health effects, two different dimensions of alcohol consumption have been shown to affect health: average volume of alcohol consumption and patterns of drinking, especially heavy drinking occasions (binge drinking). As in the previous CRA 2000 study *(76)*, patterns of drinking were used in addition to average volume in the modelling of impact on injury and ischaemic heart disease. Exposure distributions for alcohol consumption categories and drinking patterns were estimated for 2004 using large representative surveys in the 2000s and national estimates of average recorded and unrecorded adult per capita alcohol consumption for 2003, using methods described by Rehm et al. *(77)*.

The identified alcohol-attributable disease and injury conditions and relative risk estimates were the same as in the CRA 2000 *(76)* with one addition: colon and rectum cancer was added, based on the 2007 evaluation of the International Agency for Research on Cancer on the carcinogenicity of alcohol beverages *(77, 78)*.

Illicit drugs

The global burden of disease cause category "drug use disorders" includes heroin and cocaine dependence and problem use, and is therefore 100% attributed to illicit drugs. The PAFs for HIV/AIDS and hepatitis B and C due to illicit drugs were derived as described by Degenhardt et al. *(79)*. For HIV/AIDS, PAFs were updated for 2004 using country and regional estimates of transmission-mode proportions for injecting drug use; these estimates were from UNAIDS monitoring reports and other publications *(59-64)*. For the GBD 2004, estimates of deaths due to drug use disorders for 2002 were updated using regional trends in the use of illicit opiate drugs reported by the United Nations Office on Drugs and Crime *(18)*.

Unsafe water, sanitation and hygiene

Unsafe water, sanitation and hygiene is divided into six exposure categories, ranging from the ideal scenario of improved drinking water and sanitation with high population coverage, to the worst scenario of having neither. "Improved water" refers to the coverage by an improved drinking-water source, and "improved sanitation" refers to coverage by an improved sanitation facility. Improved drinking-water sources include: piped water into dwelling, plot or yard; public tap or standpipe; tubewell or borehole; protected dug well; protected spring; and rainwater collection. Improved sanitation facilities include: flush or pour-flush to piped sewer system, septic tank or pit latrine; ventilated improved pit latrine; pit latrine with slab; and composting toilet. Exposure estimates came from the WHO/UNICEF Joint Monitoring Programme for Water Supply and Sanitation; coverage data were for the year 2004 *(19)*. Relatives risks for diarrhoea were from the CRA 2000 study *(80)*.

Urban outdoor air pollution

Many air pollutants are harmful to human health; following the CRA 2000 study, we only considered the effects of particulate matter on health *(81)*. Exposure to particulate matter increases the risk of cardiopulmonary conditions, respiratory infections and lung cancer. The mean concentration of particulate matter with an aerodynamic diameter of 10 µm or less (PM_{10}) was estimated for all cities with a population over 100 000 using both modelled and measured data for the years 2002–2004, including country data reported to WHO *(81, 82)*. The proportion of PM_{10} that has an aerodynamic diameter of 2.5 µm or fewer ($PM_{2.5}$) was estimated for three regions: low-mortality European countries (0.73), developed countries (0.65) and developing countries (0.5) *(20)*. The relative risks for respiratory infections and lung cancer were from the CRA 2000 study *(81)*. The relative risks for cardiopulmonary mortality from the CRA 2000 study were used, but a revised exposure–response function (as recommended by Ostro et al. *(20)*) was used.

Indoor smoke from solid fuels

Indoor smoke exposure is measured by estimating the proportion of the population using solid fuels or coal. A ventilation factor is also calculated for countries to take into account exposure to smoke. These estimates were updated by WHO in 2007 using data from health surveys, including the World Health Survey *(83)*. The relative risks for lower respiratory infections, chronic obstructive pulmonary disease and lung cancer come from the CRA 2000 study *(84)*.

Lead exposure

New WHO estimates of blood lead levels, based on a systematic review, were used for this analysis. These estimates reflect the decline in mean blood lead levels since 2000, due to the continuing phase-out of leaded fuels. In addition to considering the effect of lead exposure during development on mild mental retardation, we considered the effect of adult exposure to lead on blood pressure, as was done in the CRA 2000 methods *(85)*, updated with the relative risks for increased blood pressure used in this analysis *(45)*. Following the CRA 2000 study, the effect of acute lead poisoning was not considered in this study. The ideal exposure level for lead is less than 1 μg/dl, however, effects are only estimated to 5 μg/dl to be consistent with available epidemiological evidence.

Climate change

The CRA 2000 study compared observed and projected climate conditions (based on several climate change scenarios) with a counterfactual situation, represented by average climate conditions during 1961–1990, when the effect of carbon emissions on climate was thought to be minimal *(86)*. We estimated the climate conditions for 2004 using projections from the original analysis. The projected climate conditions were linked to health outcomes, including malaria incidence, diarrhoea incidence, malnutrition (via the effects on yields of agricultural crops) and flooding, as described in the CRA 2000 study. Although McMichael et al. *(86)* quantified the effect of increased average temperatures on the balance of cardiovascular mortality in cold and hot temperatures, it is not known whether these deaths were brought forward or delayed by years or only a few weeks. To be consistent with analyses for other risk factors, these deaths were not included in the total deaths presented in summary tables and figures.

Occupational exposures and hazards

The CRA 2000 study included estimates of the disease and injury burden produced by selected occupational risk factors: occupational carcinogens, airborne particulates, noise, ergonomic stressors and risk factors for injuries *(87)*. The disease burden for mesothelioma attributable to asbestos exposure, and for asbestosis, silicosis and pneumoconiosis attributable to occupational exposures, were discussed by Concha-Barientos et al. *(87)*, but not included in the overall attributable mortality and disease burden estimates for occupational exposures and hazards.

PAFs from the CRA 2000 study *(87)* were assumed to apply for 2004 for the five selected occupational risks. In addition, asbestos-caused mesothelioma was also included in the 2004 estimates for occupational carcinogens: PAFs were from Driscoll et al. *(88)*. Asbestosis, silicosis and pneumoconiosis due to occupational exposures were included in the 2004 estimates for airborne particulates: PAFs were from Driscoll et al. *(89)*.

Unsafe health-care injections

Hauri et al. *(90, 91)* estimated the burden of contaminated injections in health-care settings for the year 2000. Globally, they estimated that 5% of HIV infections, 32% of hepatitis B infections and 40% of hepatitis C infections were due to inadequately sterilized injection equipment used in health-care settings. Their analysis for HIV transmission assumed an average transmission probability per contaminated injection of 1.2%, and an average of 0.3% for all needlestick injury plus 2.1% for deep needlestick injury. A more recent meta-analysis by Baggaley et al. *(92)* estimated a range of 0.24–0.65% with a point estimate of 0.45%, which we used here. This is consistent with another recent review *(93)* and an analysis of observed HIV transmission in a rural population in Uganda *(94)*.

Attributable fractions for HIV due to unsafe health-care injections were further adjusted to take account of the recent downwards revisions for HIV incidence, prevalence and mortality in many regions *(63)*. Data for India from the National AIDS Control Organisation AIDS case reporting system for 2007 gave a transmission distribution of sexual (87.4%), mother to child (4.7%), unsafe blood products (1.7%), infected needles and syringes (1.8%), and unspecified and other (4.1%) *(95)*. Making a conservative assumption that 25% of the unspecified and other transmission is from unsafe medical injections, we have assumed that the fraction of HIV incidence due to unsafe medical injections in India is 3.0%, with an uncertainty range of 1.8% to 5%.

Hauri et al. applied the same age-specific PAFs for HIV incidence and mortality *(90, 91)*. However, recent evidence suggests that incident HIV cases due to unsafe injections in the age range 0–4 years will survive at least 5 years *(96, 97)*, so PAFs for HIV/AIDS mortality have been set to zero. Mortality PAFs for ages 5–14 years were also recalculated using the incidence PAF for 0–4 years, together with estimates of the proportion of infected people who die before age 15 years.

With these revisions, the global proportion of HIV deaths attributable to unsafe medical injections was reduced to 1.3% in 2004. Use of the upper and lower bounds for the HIV PAF for India give a range of 0.9% to 1.8% for this proportion. The revised PAF for African countries with high HIV prevalence was 1.5%, which is reasonably consistent with recent estimates for Kenya and Uganda *(98, 99)*.

Child sexual abuse

The original WHO CRA study *(25)* produced estimates of the burden of disease attributable to child sexual abuse. We used those estimates for relative risks and the prevalence of child sexual abuse (based on epidemiological studies) and assumed no trend in prevalence of child sexual abuse between 2000 and 2004.

Infections and cancers

In our analysis of the primary risks for cancer, we also calculated the proportion of cancers caused by chronic infections based on prior publications *(100, 101)*. Parkin *(100)* estimated the proportion of bladder cancer caused by blood flukes; cervical cancer caused by human papillomavirus; mouth and oropharynx cancers and lymphoma caused by herpesvirus; and stomach cancer caused by *H. pylori* infection. Perz et al. *(101)* calculated the fraction of liver cancer attributed to hepatitis B and C. We applied the attributable fractions calculated by Parkin and Perz et al. to the GBD 2004 estimates of cancer incidence and mortality to estimate the contribution of infections to the cancer burden worldwide.

Table A1: Definitions, theoretical minima, disease outcomes and data sources for the selected global risk factors

Risk factor	Exposure variable	Theoretical minimum	Outcomes[a]	Exposure estimates	Hazard estimates
Childhood and maternal undernutrition					
Underweight	Children < −1 SD weight-for-age compared with the new WHO standards in 1 SD increments (37, 38); maternal body mass index <20 kg/m²	Same proportion of children below −1 SD weight-for-age as the international reference group; all women of childbearing age with body mass index ≥20 kg/m²	Mortality and acute morbidity from diarrhoeal diseases, malaria, measles, pneumonia and selected other infectious diseases and protein-energy malnutrition for children <5; perinatal conditions from maternal underweight	Updated estimates of childhood underweight prevalence in 2005 according to new WHO standards (35–38). Updated estimates of maternal underweight for WHO Member States (39)	Revised relative risks for child underweight and IUGR outcomes (9)
Iron deficiency	Haemoglobin concentrations estimated from prevalence of anaemia	Haemoglobin distributions that halve anaemia prevalence in malarial regions and reduce it by 60% in non-malarial regions, estimated to occur if all iron deficiency were eliminated[b]	Anaemia and its sequelae (including cognitive impairment), maternal mortality	Updated estimates for WHO Member States (11)	Systematic review and meta-analysis of cohort studies (41)
Vitamin A deficiency	Prevalence of vitamin A deficiency, estimated as low serum retinol concentrations (<0.70 μmol/l) among children aged 0–4 years	No vitamin A deficiency	Mortality due to diarrhoeal diseases, measles, prematurity and low birth weight, and neonatal infections (children <5), morbidity due to vitamin A deficiency and its sequelae (all age groups)	Updated estimates of the prevalence of vitamin A deficiency in children <5 for 2004 (9)	From Rice et al. (42) for 6–59 months, new relative risk estimates for 0–5 months (9)
Zinc deficiency	Less than the USA recommended dietary allowances for zinc	No zinc deficiency	Diarrhoeal diseases, pneumonia, malaria	Updated estimates of the prevalence of zinc deficiency in children <5 for 2004 (9)	New relative risk estimates from intervention trials (9)
Suboptimal breastfeeding	Prevalence of suboptimal breast-feeding (exclusive, predominant, partial, non-breastfeeding)	100% exclusive breastfeeding from 0–5 months and any breastfeeding from 6–23 months	Diarrhoeal diseases, lower respiratory infections, other causes arising in perinatal period (infectious disease component only)	New estimates of prevalence of suboptimal breastfeeding from recent national survey data (9, 43, 44)	New relative risk estimates from a random effects meta-analysis of 7 studies, including a multicentre study in Ghana, India and Peru (9)
Other nutrition-related risk factors and physical activity					
High blood pressure	Usual level of systolic blood pressure	Mean of 115 mmHg and SD of 6 mmHg	IHD, stroke, hypertensive disease and other cardiovascular diseases	Updated WHO estimates for Member States (39)	Meta-analysis of 61 cohort studies with 1 million North American and European participants (45)

(Table A1 continued)

Risk factor	Exposure variable	Theoretical minimum	Outcomes[a]	Exposure estimates	Hazard estimates
High cholesterol	Usual level of total blood cholesterol	Mean of 3.8 mmol/l and standard deviation of 0.6 mmol/l	IHD, ischaemic stroke	Updated WHO estimates for Member States (39)	Meta-analysis of 61 cohorts with 900 000 participants from Europe and North America (28)
Overweight and obesity (high BMI)	BMI (height (m) divided by weight (kg) squared)	Mean of 21 kg/m² and standard deviation of 1 kg/m²	IHD, ischaemic stroke, hypertensive disease, diabetes, osteoarthritis, colon and uterine cancers, post-menopausal breast cancer	Updated WHO estimates for Member States (39)	APCS meta-analysis for cardiovascular and metabolic outcomes (47) and new meta-analysis of 221 data sets for cancers (46)
High blood glucose	Fasting plasma glucose (FPG) concentration	Mean of 4.9 mmol/l and standard deviation of 0.3 mmol/l	Diabetes mellitus, IHD, cerebrovascular disease	Regional estimates of FPG distribution for people aged 30 years and over (8)	APCS meta-analysis of 13 cohorts with 200 000 par-ticipants from the Asia-Pacific region (57)
Low fruit and vegetable consumption	Fruit and vegetable intake per day	600g (SD 50 g) intake per day for adults	IHD, stroke, colon and rectum cancers, gastric cancer, lung cancer, oesophageal cancer	Systematic review of food consumption surveys and food availability data (49)	Systematic review and meta-analyses of published cohort studies (49, 51-53)
Physical inactivity	Four categories of inactive, low, medium, and high activity levels (50, 55). Activity in discretionary-time, work and transport considered	High activity level: minimum 3 days per week of vigorous intensity activity (minimum 1500 MET-minutes/week), or 7 days per week of any intensity activity (minimum 3000 MET-minutes/week)	IHD, breast cancer, colon cancer, diabetes mellitus	Prevalence estimates for three categories of physical inactivity from Bull et al. (54). Sufficiently active category split into moder-ate and highly active using data for 28 countries (50, 56).	Systematic review of published cohort studies (50, 54)
Sexual and reproductive health					
Unsafe sex	Sex with an infected partner without any measures to prevent infection	No unsafe sex	HIV/AIDS, sexually transmitted infections and cervical cancer	PAF = 1 (STDs excluding HIV/AIDS, cervical cancer); HIV/AIDS proportions from UNAIDS Reference Group estimates (58), updated using information from UNAIDS Monitoring Reports and other sources (59-64)	
Lack of contraception	Prevalence of traditional meth-ods or non-use of contraception	Use of modern contraceptives for all women who want to space or limit future pregnancies	Maternal mortality and morbidity	Data from World contraceptive use 2007 (67)	From CRA 2000 study (66)

(Table A1 continued)

Risk factor	Exposure variable	Theoretical minimum	Outcomes[a]	Exposure estimates	Hazard estimates
Addictive substances					
Tobacco	Current levels of smoking impact ratio (indirect indicator of accumulated smoking risk based on excess lung cancer mortality); oral tobacco use prevalence	No tobacco use	Lung, upper aerodigestive, stomach, liver, pancreas, cervix, bladder, colon, rectum and kidney cancers, myeloid leukaemia, COPD, other respiratory diseases, tuberculosis, all vascular diseases, diabetes	Updated smoking impact ratios calculated from GBD 2004 lung cancer mortality estimates (2); oral tobacco prevalence for South Asia from WHS–India (70)	Relative risks for most causes from the ACS cohort (69, 71, 72), as used by Danaei et al. (50); from meta-analyses for tuberculosis (73) and for mouth and oropharynx cancers from chewing tobacco (74)
Alcohol	Current alcohol consumption volumes and patterns	No alcohol use	IHD, stroke, hypertensive disease, diabetes, liver cancer, mouth and oropharynx cancer, breast cancer, oesophagus cancer, colon and rectum cancers, other cancers, liver cirrhosis, epilepsy, alcohol use disorders, depression, intentional and unintentional injuries	Updated estimates of alcohol consumption for WHO Member States (75, 77).	Relative risks for colon and rectum cancer added (78); other relative risks from Rehm et al. (76)
Illicit drugs	Use of amphetamine, cocaine, heroin or other opioids and intravenous drug use	No illicit drug use	HIV/AIDS, overdose, drug use disorder, suicide, and trauma	Revised based on trends in illicit drug use reported by UNODC (18)	PAFs from Degenhardt et al. (79); HIV/AIDS PAFs updated using information from UNAIDS Monitoring Reports and other sources (59–64)
Environmental risks					
Indoor smoke from solid fuels	Use of solid fuel or coal household use taking into account a ventilation factor	No solid fuel or coal use	Lower respiratory infections, lung cancer, COPD	Updated estimates for WHO Member States (83)	Relative risks come from the CRA 2000 study (84)
Unsafe water, sanitation and hygiene	Six categories of exposure: • Ideal situation, corresponding to the absence of transmission of diarrhoeal disease through water, sanitation and hygiene • Regulated water supply and partial sewage treatment • Improved water and basic sanitation • Basic sanitation only • Improved water only • No improved supply or basic sanitation	Absence of transmission of diarrhoeal disease through water and sanitation	Diarrhoeal diseases	Updated estimates for WHO Member States (19)	Relative risks come from the CRA 2000 study (80)

1

2

3

Annex A

References

(Table A1 continued)

Risk factor	Exposure variable	Theoretical minimum	Outcomes[a]	Exposure estimates	Hazard estimates
Urban outdoor air pollution	Annual mean fine particulate matter with an aerodynamic diameter greater than 2.5 µm ($PM_{2.5}$) and 10 µm (PM_{10})	Mean concentration of 7.5 µg/m³ for $PM_{2.5}$ and 15 µg/m³ for PM_{10}	Respiratory infections, lung cancers, selected cardiopulmonary diseases	Updated estimates for WHO Member States (81, 82)	Relative risks come from the CRA 2000 study (81)
Lead exposure	Mean and standard deviation of blood lead level	Blood lead below 1 µg/dl[c]	Mild mental retardation, raised blood pressure (which increases the risk of IHD), stroke, hypertensive disease and other cardiovascular diseases	Updated WHO estimates for Member States	Relative risks for mild mental retardation and raised blood pressure from the CRA 2000 study (85); relative risks for the effect of blood pressure on cardiovascular outcomes from the prospective cohorts study (45)
Global climate change	Climate scenarios based on actual and counterfactual carbon emissions and concentrations	Average of 1961–1990 climate conditions	Diarrhoea, flood injury, malaria, undernutrition and associated disease outcomes	Climate change that resulted from unmitigated carbon emissions, as projected to 2004 in the 2000 CRA study (86)	Relative risks derived from observed relationships between climate and health, from CRA 2000 study (86)
Occupational risks					
Occupational risk factors for injuries	Current proportions of workers exposed to injury risk factors	Exposure corresponding to lowest rate of work-related fatalities observed: 1 per million per year for 16- to 17-year-olds employed as service workers in the USA	Unintentional injuries	PAFs estimated for CRA 2000 assumed to hold for 2004 (87)	
Occupational carcinogens	Proportions of workers exposed to background, low, and high levels of workplace carcinogens	No work-related exposure above background to chemical or physical agents that cause cancer	Leukaemia, lung cancer, mesothelioma	PAFs estimated for CRA 2000 assumed to hold for 2004 (87); PAFs for mesothelioma are from Driscoll et al. (88)	
Occupational airborne particulates	Proportions of workers with background, low and high levels of exposure	No work-related exposure above background	COPD and asthma, pneumoconiosis, silicosis and asbestosis	PAFs estimated for CRA 2000 assumed to hold for 2004 (87); PAFs for asbestosis, silicosis and pneumoconioses are from Driscoll et al. (89)	
Occupational ergonomic stressors	High, moderate, and low exposure based on occupational categories	Physical workload at the level of managers and professionals (low)	Lower back pain	PAFs estimated for CRA 2000 assumed to hold for 2004 (87)	

(Table A1 continued)

Risk factor	Exposure variable	Theoretical minimum	Outcomes[a]	Exposure estimates	Hazard estimates
Occupational noise	High and moderate exposure categories (>90 dBA and 85–90 dBA)	Less than 85 dBA on average over 8 working hours	Hearing loss	PAFs estimated for CRA 2000 assumed to hold for 2004 (87)	
Other selected risks					
Unsafe health-care injections	Exposure to at least one contaminated injection	No contaminated injections	Acute infection with HBV, HCV and HIV, cirrhosis and liver cancer	Previous PAFs for HIV (90) adjusted to take into account a recent meta-analysis of the transmission probability for HIV through reuse of a contaminated needle (92), revised estimates for HIV incidence and prevalence (63) and recent data on transmission modes for HIV infection in India (95). Previous PAFs for hepatitis B and C, cirrhosis and liver cancer assumed to apply for 2004.	
Childhood sexual abuse	Prevalence of non-contact abuse, contact abuse and intercourse	No abuse	Depression, panic disorder, alcohol abuse/dependence, drug abuse/dependence, post-traumatic stress disorder and suicide in adulthood	Prevalences estimated by Andrews et al. for year 2000 assumed to apply for 2004 (25)	Systematic review and meta-analysis of published studies (25)

ACS, American Cancer Society; AIDS, acquired immunodeficiency syndrome; BMI, body mass index; COPD, chronic obstructive pulmonary disease; CRA, comparative risk assessment; dBA, A-weighted decibels; (the noise power calculated in dB); GBD, global burden of disease; HIV, human immunodeficiency virus; HBV, hepatitis B virus; HCV, hepatitis C virus; IHD, ischaemic heart disease; IUGR, intrauterine growth restriction; MET, metabolic equivalent; PAF, population attributable fraction; PM, particulate matter; SD, standard deviation; STD, sexually transmitted disease; UNAIDS, Joint United Nations Programme on HIV/AIDS; UNODC, United Nations Office on Drugs and Crime; USA, United States of America; WHO, World Health Organization; WHS, World Health Survey.

a Outcomes likely to be causal but not quantified due to lack of sufficient evidence on prevalence and/or hazard size are not listed here.

b The theoretical minimum haemoglobin levels vary across regions and age-sex groups (from 11.66 g/dl in children under 5 years in South-East Asian Region (SEAR)-D to > 14.5 g/dl in adult males in developed countries) because the other risks for anaemia (e.g. malaria) vary.

c Theoretical minimum for lead is the blood lead level expected at background exposure levels. Health effects were quantified for blood lead levels above 5 μg/dl where epidemiological studies have quantified hazards.

Table A2: Summary prevalence of selected risk factors by income group in WHO regions,[a] 2004

Risk factor	Prevalence measure[b]	World			Africa	South-East Asia	The Americas		
		Both sexes	Males	Females	Low and middle income	Low and middle income	Total	High income	Low and middle income
Population (millions)		6 437	3 244	3 193	738	1 672	874	329	545
		(000)	*(000)*	*(000)*	*(000)*	*(000)*	*(000)*	*(000)*	*(000)*
Childhood and maternal undernutrition									
Underweight	Child stunting (%)[c]	29	29	29	43	42	12	2	16
	Child wasting (%)[d]	9	9	9	11	15	2	1	2
Iron deficiency	Prevalence of iron-deficiency anaemia (%)[e]								
	Children aged 0–14 years	26	26	26	34	41	12	2	16
	Adults aged ≥15 years	15	12	18	21	21	6	3	8
	Pregnant women	–	–	41	56	48	24	5	31
Vitamin A deficiency	Children at risk of vitamin A deficiency (%)[f]	64	64	64	93	92	20	0	28
Zinc deficiency	Children living in zinc-deficient areas (%)[g]	89	89	88	100	100	66	1	91
Suboptimal breastfeeding	Not exclusively breastfed to 6 months (%)	69	69	69	78	62	68	61	71
Other nutrition-related risk factors and physical activity									
High blood pressure	Mean systolic pressure (mmHg)[h]	126.5	126.9	126.0	128.2	125.3	125.6	126.3	125.0
	Systolic ≥140 mmHg (%)[h]	23	22	23	27	19	21	21	21
High cholesterol	Mean serum cholesterol (mmol/l)[i]	5.1	5.0	5.1	4.3	5.1	5.3	5.4	5.3
	Cholesterol level ≥6 mmol/l[i]	22	20	23	8	21	28	28	28
High blood glucose	Mean fasting plasma glucose (mmol/l)[j]	5.4	5.4	5.4	5.1	5.6	5.4	5.4	5.3
	Diabetic (fpg >7 mmol/l) (%)[j]	11	11	11	4	17	10	13	9
Overweight and obesity	Mean BMI (kg/m²)[k]	24.5	24.3	24.6	23.0	22.1	27.9	29.0	27.0
	Overweight and obese (BMI ≥ 25) (%)	42	40	43	30	22	70	76	65
	Obese (BMI ≥ 30) (%)	12	9	15	6	2	33	43	26
Low fruit and vegetable intake	Mean fruit and vegetable intake (g/day)[l]	303	314	293	279	239	244	297	207
	Less than five servings per day[m]	67	64	71	71	80	69	65	71
Physical inactivity	Inactive (%)	17	16	19	11	16	22	21	22
	Insufficiently active (%)	41	42	39	49	38	38	41	36
	Moderately active (%)	17	15	20	14	17	19	20	18
	Highly active (%)	25	28	22	25	28	21	18	24
Addictive substances									
Tobacco use	Current smokers (%)[l]	26	43	10	9	21	24	23	26
	Smoking impact ratio (%)[l]	18	25	10	5	12	25	40	13
Alcohol use	Proportion consuming alcohol (%)[l]	44	55	34	36	12	65	58	69
	≥40 grams alcohol/day (%)[l]	13	22	3	18	5	16	19	14
	Average per capita consumption (grams alcohol per day)[l]	14	21	6	16	4	19	21	18
Sexual and reproductive health									
Unmet contraceptive need	Unmet need (%)[n]	43	0	43	70	39	23	2	34
Environmental risks									
Unsafe water, sanitation, hygiene	Improved water supply (%)[o]	83	83	83	57	84	94	100	91
	Improved sanitation (%)[p]	59	59	60	40	41	86	100	77
Urban outdoor air pollution	Concentration of particles less 10 µm (µg/m³)	62	62	61	65	92	36	24	47
Indoor smoke from solid fuels	Proportion using biofuel (%)	46	46	45	77	81	11	0	18

Risk factor	Prevalence measure[b]	Eastern Mediterranean			Europe			Western Pacific		
		Total	High income	Low and middle income	Total	High income	Low and middle income	Total	High income	Low and middle income
Population (millions)		520	31	489	883	407	476	1 738	204	1 534
		(000)	(000)	(000)	(000)	(000)	(000)	(000)	(000)	(000)
Childhood and maternal undernutrition										
Underweight	Child stunting (%) [c]	29	16	30	8	2	13	18	4	19
	Child wasting (%) [d]	10	3	11	2	1	3	5	1	6
Iron deficiency	Prevalence of iron-deficiency anaemia (%) [e]									
	Children aged 0–14 years	24	15	24	12	5	17	16	7	17
	Adults aged ≥15 years	13	10	13	8	6	10	15	9	16
	Pregnant women	44	31	44	25	14	32	30	17	32
Vitamin A deficiency	Children at risk of vitamin A deficiency (%) [f]	78	33	81	16	1	27	33	8	35
Zinc deficiency	Children living in zinc-deficient areas (%) [g]	100	99	100	28	3	46	94	28	100
Suboptimal breastfeeding	Not exclusively breastfed to 6 months (%)	72	87	71	66	62	68	71	68	71
Other nutrition-related risk factors and physical activity										
High blood pressure	Mean systolic pressure (mmHg) [h]	126.8	123.8	127.1	133.7	134.0	133.4	123.1	129.2	122.0
	Systolic ≥140 mmHg (%) [h]	23	17	23	36	36	35	19	28	17
High cholesterol	Mean serum cholesterol (mmol/l) [i]	4.8	4.8	4.8	5.5	5.7	5.4	4.9	5.4	4.9
	Cholesterol level ≥6 mmol/l [i]	15	15	15	34	39	29	17	26	16
High blood glucose	Mean fasting plasma glucose (mmol/l) [j]	5.6	5.5	5.6	5.4	5.5	5.3	5.3	5.5	5.3
	Diabetic (fpg >7 mmol/l) (%) [j]	17	15	17	12	14	9	7	14	6
Overweight and obesity	Mean BMI (kg/m²) [k]	25.2	28.5	25.0	26.9	26.8	27.0	23.4	24.1	23.3
	Overweight and obese (BMI ≥ 25) (%)	48	74	46	65	65	65	31	39	30
	Obese (BMI ≥ 30) (%)	18	37	16	24	23	25	3	7	2
Low fruit and vegetable intake	Mean fruit and vegetable intake (g/day) [l]	350	343	350	376	462	298	343	399	335
	Less than five servings per day [m]	58	59	57	56	42	69	64	52	66
Physical inactivity	Inactive (%)	17	18	17	20	18	22	16	17	16
	Insufficiently active (%)	37	38	37	43	51	35	41	49	40
	Moderately active (%)	18	18	18	18	17	19	17	17	17
	Highly active (%)	27	26	28	20	15	24	26	17	27
Addictive substances										
Tobacco use	Current smokers (%) [i]	18	18	18	33	29	37	32	29	32
	Smoking impact ratio (%) [i]	12	1	13	36	32	40	12	17	11
Alcohol use	Proportion consuming alcohol (%) [i]	6	10	6	74	83	66	58	73	56
	≥40 grams alcohol/day (%) [i]	1	1	1	27	25	28	11	14	11
	Average per capita consumption (grams alcohol per day) [i]	2	2	1	26	27	25	15	19	15
Sexual and reproductive health										
Unmet contraceptive need	Unmet need (%) [n]	52	50	52	20	0	35	53	7	58
Environmental risks										
Unsafe water, sanitation, hygiene	Improved water supply (%) [o]	85	92	85	96	100	92	80	94	78
	Improved sanitation (%) [p]	67	90	65	92	100	86	52	87	47
Urban outdoor air pollution	Concentration of particles less 10 µm (µg/m³)	116	98	118	35	30	39	67	34	76
Indoor smoke from solid fuels	Proportion using biofuel (%)	41	0	43	6	0	11	37	0	42

(Table A2 continued)

Risk factor	Prevalence measure[b]	World			Africa	South-East Asia	The Americas		
		Both sexes	Males	Females	Low and middle income	Low and middle income	Total	High income	Low and middle income
Population (millions)		6 437	3 244	3 193	738	1 672	874	329	545
		(000)	(000)	(000)	(000)	(000)	(000)	(000)	(000)
Other selected risks									
Unsafe health-care injections	Proportion receiving injections contaminated with hepatitis B per year (%)	6	6	6	4	9	0	0	0
Child sexual abuse	Proportion of adults with history of abuse (%) [q]	16	10	22	15	26	8	11	6

a See Table A5 for a list of Member States by WHO region and income category.

b Estimates are for the population most relevant to the risk factor – alcohol, childhood sexual abuse, physical inactivity are for ages ≥15 years; blood pressure, cholesterol, overweight, and fruit and vegetables are for ages ≥30 years; iron, vitamin A, zinc and underweight are for children under 5 years; and lack of contraception is for females 15–44 years. Many risk factors were characterized at multiple levels for the analyses in this report – this table does not include full details of exposure distributions but rather selected informative indicators (eg. % exposed, % exceeding a commonly used threshold, mean level).

c Prevalence of stunting here defined as height-for-age more than 2 standard deviations below the WHO reference standard for children aged 0–4 years. Health outcomes were assessed for levels of stunting more than 1 standard deviation below the WHO reference standard.

d Prevalence of wasting here defined as weight-for-age more than 2 standard deviations below the WHO reference standard for children aged 0–4 years.

e Prevalence of anaemia attributed to iron-deficiency only. Anaemia is defined as blood haemoglobin level <110 g/l in pregnant women, <120 g/l in children and adult women and <130 g/l in adult men. Attributable deaths and DALYs are calculated using the estimated distribution of blood haemoglobin among those who have anaemia.

f Prevalences were estimated based on the per cent of children under five years of age living in areas classified as vitamin A deficient based on population survey data for low plasma or tissue retinol levels and xerophthalmia, together with information on coverage of vitamin A supplementation programs (9).

g Child populations of countries were classified as at risk of zinc deficiency based on the prevalence of stunting and the adequacy of absorbable zinc in the food supply at the country level (9).

h Persons aged ≥30 years.

i For persons aged ≥ 30 years. 1 mmol/l = 38.7 mg/dl; 6 mmol/l = 232 mg/dl.

j For persons aged ≥30 years. 5.55 mmol/l = 100 mg/dl; 7 mmol/l = 125 mg/dl.

k For persons aged ≥30 years. Body mass index (BMI) is defined as weight (kg) divided by height (m) squared.

l Persons aged ≥15 years.

m Persons aged ≥15 years. Average serving assumed to correspond to 80 g.

n Proportion of women who want to prevent or space conception and are not using modern contraceptive methods.

o Proportion of the population with improved or regulated water supply.

p Proportion of the population with improved sanitation coverage or full sewage treatment.

q Proportion of adults aged ≥ 15 years reporting a history of child sexual abuse by an older person involving contact (genital touching or fondling), intercourse or attempted intercourse.

Risk factor	Prevalence measure[b]	Eastern Mediterranean			Europe			Western Pacific		
		Total	High income	Low and middle income	Total	High income	Low and middle income	Total	High income	Low and middle income
Population (millions)		520	31	489	883	407	476	1 738	204	1 534
		(000)	(000)	(000)	(000)	(000)	(000)	(000)	(000)	(000)
Other selected risks										
Unsafe health-care injections	Proportion receiving injections contaminated with hepatitis B per year (%)	9	0	9	0	0	1	7	0	8
Child sexual abuse	Proportion of adults with history of abuse (%) [q]	12	11	12	10	8	12	16	13	16

1

2

3

Annex A

References

Table A3: Attributable mortality by risk factor and income group in WHO regions,[a] estimates for 2004

Risk factor[b]	Sex						Africa	South-East Asia	The Americas		
	Both sexes		Males		Females		Low and middle income	Low and middle income	Total	High income	Low and middle income
Population (millions)	6 437		3 244		3 193		738	1 672	874	329	545
	(000)	% total	(000)	% total	(000)	% total	(000)	(000)	(000)	(000)	(000)
Total deaths (all causes)	58 772	100	31 082	100	27 690	100	11 248	15 279	6 58	695	3 464
Childhood and maternal undernutrition											
Underweight	2 225	3.8	1 163	3.7	1 062	3.8	982	829	27	0	27
Iron deficiency	273	0.5	55	0.2	217	0.8	87	122	18	3	15
Vitamin A deficiency	651	1.1	339	1.1	312	1.1	273	252	10	0	10
Zinc deficiency	433	0.7	226	0.7	208	0.7	249	111	8	0	8
Suboptimal breastfeeding	1 247	2.1	649	2.1	599	2.2	479	366	67	5	62
Other nutrition-related risk factors and physical activity											
High blood pressure	7 512	12.8	3 544	11.4	3 968	14.3	515	1 438	828	412	416
High cholesterol	2 625	4.5	1 371	4.4	1 255	4.5	83	756	338	174	164
High blood glucose	3 387	5.8	1 675	5.4	1 712	6.2	241	1 044	501	212	289
Overweight and obesity	2 825	4.8	1 319	4.2	1 506	5.4	166	343	587	288	299
Low fruit and vegetable intake	1 674	2.8	898	2.9	777	2.8	89	450	183	82	102
Physical inactivity	3 219	5.5	1 567	5.0	1 651	6.0	202	782	451	229	222
Addictive substances											
Tobacco use	5 110	8.7	3 578	11.5	1 532	5.5	145	1 037	863	600	263
Alcohol use	2 252	3.8	1 942	6.2	310	1.1	269	354	347	56	291
Illicit drug use	245	0.4	192	0.6	53	0.2	9	73	31	16	14
Sexual and reproductive health											
Unsafe sex	2 355	4.0	1 033	3.3	1 321	4.8	1 746	332	107	20	87
Unmet contraceptive need[c]	163	0.3	0	0.0	163	0.6	60	73	6	0	6
Environmental risks											
Unsafe water, sanitation, hygiene	1 908	3.2	994	3.2	914	3.3	896	599	59	0	6
Urban outdoor air pollution	1 152	2.0	609	2.0	543	2.0	61	207	143	72	71
Indoor smoke from solid fuels	1 965	3.3	886	2.9	1 079	3.9	551	630	30	0	29
Lead exposure	143	0.2	94	0.3	49	0.2	9	70	7	0	6
Global climate change	141	0.2	73	0.2	68	0.2	57	58	2	0	2
Occupational risks											
Risk factors for injuries	352	0.6	331	1.1	21	0.1	42	121	24	3	20
Carcinogens	177	0.3	137	0.4	41	0.1	6	32	19	10	9
Airborne particulates	457	0.8	352	1.1	105	0.4	29	118	29	15	14
Ergonomic stressors	1	0.0	1	0.0	0	0.0	0	0	0	0	0
Noise	0	0.0	0	0.0	0	0.0	0	0	0	0	0
Other selected risks											
Unsafe health care injections	417	0.7	279	0.9	138	0.5	30	121	2	0	2
Child sexual abuse	82	0.1	41	0.1	41	0.1	4	38	4	2	2

[a] See Table A5 for a list of Member States by WHO region and income category.
[b] The table shows estimated deaths attributable to each risk factor considered individually, relative to its own counterfactual risk exposure distribution. These risks may act in part through, or jointly with, other risks. Total deaths attributable to groups of risk factors will thus usually be less than the sum of the deaths attributable to individual risks.
[c] Unmet contraceptive need refers to "non-use and use of ineffective methods of contraception" among those wanting to control their fertility to avoid conception or space the birth of children.

Risk factor[b]	Eastern Mediterranean			Europe			Western Pacific		
	Total	High income	Low and middle income	Total	High income	Low and middle income	Total	High income	Low and middle income
Population (millions)	520	31	489	883	407	476	1 738	204	1 534
	(000)	(000)	(000)	(000)	(000)	(000)	(000)	(000)	(000)
Total deaths (all causes)	4 306	113	4 194	9 493	3 809	5 683	12 191	1 478	10 714
Childhood and maternal undernutrition									
Underweight	301	1	300	28	0	27	59	0	58
Iron deficiency	25	0	25	8	4	4	12	1	11
Vitamin A deficiency	86	1	86	10	0	10	20	0	19
Zinc deficiency	46	0	46	5	0	5	15	0	15
Suboptimal breastfeeding	208	2	205	36	2	33	92	1	92
Other nutrition-related risk factors and physical activity									
High blood pressure	475	19	456	2 491	740	1 752	1 764	200	1 564
High cholesterol	178	6	172	926	242	684	345	52	293
High blood glucose	283	13	270	748	258	490	570	86	484
Overweight and obesity	233	18	215	1 081	318	763	414	56	358
Low fruit and vegetable intake	78	3	75	423	77	346	451	40	412
Physical inactivity	219	8	211	992	301	691	573	87	486
Addictive substances									
Tobacco use	187	3	184	1 472	595	877	1 405	261	1 144
Alcohol use	22	1	21	618	25	593	641	52	590
Illicit drug use	47	1	46	45	11	33	41	3	38
Sexual and reproductive health									
Unsafe sex	52	0	52	54	16	38	65	6	58
Unmet contraceptive need[c]	21	0	21	1	0	1	3	0	3
Environmental risks									
Unsafe water, sanitation, hygiene	226	0	21	33	0	1	95	0	3
Urban outdoor air pollution	95	4	91	225	76	149	421	47	373
Indoor smoke from solid fuels	142	0	142	20	0	19	591	0	591
Lead exposure	26	1	25	8	0	8	23	0	22
Global climate change	20	0	20	1	0	1	4	0	4
Occupational risks									
Risk factors for injuries	43	2	42	27	4	24	95	4	91
Carcinogens	6	0	6	42	14	27	72	9	62
Airborne particulates	15	0	15	46	19	27	220	9	211
Ergonomic stressors	0	0	0	0	0	0	0	0	0
Noise	0	0	0	0	0	0	0	0	0
Other selected risks									
Unsafe health-care injections	55	0	55	14	0	14	195	9	185
Child sexual abuse	4	0	4	7	2	6	24	3	21

Table A4: Attributable DALYs by risk factor and income group in WHO regions,[a] estimates for 2004

Risk factor[b]	Sex						Africa	South-East Asia	The Americas		
	Both sexes		Males		Females		Low and middle income	Low and middle income	Total	High income	Low and middle income
Population (millions)	6 437		3 244		3 193		738	1 672	874	329	545
	(000)	% total	(000)	% total	(000)	% total	(000)	(000)	(000)	(000)	(000)
Total DALYs (all causes)	1 523 259	100	79 133	100	727 126	100	376 525	44 979	143 233	45 116	98 116
Childhood and maternal undernutrition											
Underweight	90 683	6.0	47 171	5.9	43 511	6.0	38 575	34 342	1 378	25	1 352
Iron deficiency	19 734	1.3	6 918	0.9	12 815	1.8	4 710	7 946	1 069	123	946
Vitamin A deficiency	22 099	1.5	11 499	1.4	10 600	1.5	9 323	8 548	343	0	343
Zinc deficiency	15 580	1.0	8 120	1.0	7 460	1.0	8 964	3 928	319	1	317
Suboptimal breastfeeding	43 842	2.9	22 721	2.9	21 121	2.9	16 692	12 809	2 472	187	2 285
Other nutrition-related risk factors and physical activity											
High blood pressure	57 227	3.8	30 823	3.9	26 404	3.6	5 010	13 447	5 476	2 229	3 247
High cholesterol	29 723	2.0	17 576	2.2	12 147	1.7	1 071	9 856	3 595	1 593	2 002
High blood glucose	41 305	2.7	21 468	2.7	19 837	2.7	2 906	13 326	6 166	2 374	3 792
Overweight and obesity	35 796	2.3	17 747	2.2	18 049	2.5	2 259	5 133	7 880	3 631	4 249
Low fruit and vegetable intake	15 974	1.0	9 171	1.2	6 803	0.9	1 031	4 865	1 705	674	1 031
Physical inactivity	32 099	2.1	16 795	2.1	15 304	2.1	2 289	9 010	4 349	1 913	2 435
Addictive substances											
Tobacco use	56 897	3.7	43 291	5.4	13 606	1.9	1 930	12 764	8 837	5 681	3 157
Alcohol use	69 424	4.6	59 283	7.4	10 141	1.4	7 759	12 066	13 102	3 402	9 700
Illicit drug use	13 223	0.9	10 178	1.3	3 045	0.4	1 131	2 585	3 110	1 433	1 677
Sexual and reproductive health											
Unsafe sex	70 017	4.6	30 064	3.8	39 954	5.5	50 771	10 559	3 146	536	2 610
Unmet contraceptive need[c]	11 501	0.8	0	0.0	11 501	1.6	3 645	4 934	773	6	766
Environmental risks											
Unsafe water, sanitation, hygiene	64 240	4.2	33 459	4.2	30 781	4.2	28 700	20 176	2 219	6	766
Urban outdoor air pollution	8 747	0.6	4 981	0.6	3 766	0.5	881	1 911	884	393	492
Indoor smoke from solid fuels	41 009	2.7	20 614	2.6	20 395	2.8	18 057	12 492	735	5	730
Lead exposure	8 977	0.6	4 891	0.6	4 087	0.6	1 050	4 044	580	20	560
Global climate change	5 404	0.4	2 800	0.4	2 604	0.4	2 029	2 320	81	2	80
Occupational risks											
Risk factors for injuries	11 612	0.8	10 810	1.4	802	0.1	1 385	4 029	772	95	677
Carcinogens	1 897	0.1	1 419	0.2	479	0.1	87	391	181	81	100
Airborne particulates	6 751	0.4	5 272	0.7	1 479	0.2	553	1 820	590	251	339
Ergonomic stressors	898	0.1	530	0.1	368	0.1	102	261	87	28	59
Noise	4 509	0.3	3 069	0.4	1 441	0.2	381	1 574	314	123	191
Other selected risks											
Unsafe health-care injections	6 960	0.5	4 506	0.6	2 453	0.3	827	2 308	40	0	39
Child sexual abuse	9 018	0.6	3 433	0.4	5 585	0.8	603	4 048	753	401	352

DALY, disability-adjusted life year.

a   See Table A5 for a list of Member States by WHO region and income category.

b   The table shows estimated DALYs attributable to each risk factor considered individually, relative to its own counterfactual risk exposure distribution. These risks may act in part through, or jointly, with other risks. Total DALYs attributable to groups of risk factors will thus usually be less than the sum of the DALYs attributable to individual risks.

c   Unmet contraceptive need refers to "non-use and use of ineffective methods of contraception" among those wanting to control their fertility to avoid conception or space the birth of children.

Risk factor[b]	Eastern Mediterranean			Europe			Western Pacific		
	Total	High income	Low and middle income	Total	High income	Low and middle income	Total	High income	Low and middle income
Population (millions)	520	31	489	883	407	476	1 738	204	1 534
	(000)	(000)	(000)	(000)	(000)	(000)	(000)	(000)	(000)
Total DALYs (all causes)	141 993	4 379	137 614	151 461	49 331	102 130	264 772	22 305	242 466
Childhood and maternal undernutrition									
Underweight	11 882	65	11 816	1 148	19	1 129	3 358	32	3 326
Iron deficiency	1 689	49	1 640	948	251	696	3 373	210	3 162
Vitamin A deficiency	2 915	17	2 898	318	1	317	653	4	649
Zinc deficiency	1 638	12	1 626	174	1	174	557	2	555
Suboptimal breastfeeding	7 299	89	7 210	1 263	98	1 164	3 307	36	3 270
Other nutrition-related risk factors and physical activity									
High blood pressure	4 317	188	4 129	17 121	3 807	13 314	11 856	1 273	10 583
High cholesterol	2 297	105	2 192	8 975	1 859	7 116	3 930	570	3 360
High blood glucose	3 880	258	3 623	7 304	2 308	4 996	7 722	1 077	6 645
Overweight and obesity	3 231	321	2 910	11 758	3 132	8 625	5 536	839	4 698
Low fruit and vegetable intake	908	38	870	3 624	547	3 077	3 841	299	3 542
Physical inactivity	2 612	144	2 468	8 264	2 189	6 075	5 575	806	4 768
Addictive substances									
Tobacco use	2 793	31	2 762	17 725	5 526	12 199	12 848	1 871	10 976
Alcohol use	763	53	710	17 342	3 165	14 177	18 393	1 541	16 851
Illicit drug use	2 117	22	2 095	2 395	937	1 458	1 886	155	1 731
Sexual and reproductive health									
Unsafe sex	2 166	36	2 131	1 543	384	1 159	1 832	125	1 707
Unmet contraceptive need[c]	1 671	33	1 638	131	4	127	348	4	344
Environmental risks									
Unsafe water, sanitation, hygiene	7 364	33	1 638	1 182	4	127	4 599	4	344
Urban outdoor air pollution	971	37	933	1 456	369	1 087	2 644	231	2 414
Indoor smoke from solid fuels	4 239	0	4 239	485	4	482	5 001	2	4 999
Lead exposure	1 638	91	1 547	134	7	126	1 531	11	1 521
Global climate change	756	11	745	26	1	25	192	3	190
Occupational risks									
Risk factors for injuries	1 686	63	1 623	823	114	709	2 918	115	2 803
Carcinogens	84	4	80	408	116	291	747	75	671
Airborne particulates	357	12	345	676	284	392	2 755	163	2 592
Ergonomic stressors	61	3	58	99	32	67	289	23	266
Noise	346	22	324	538	161	376	1 356	86	1 270
Other selected risks									
Unsafe health-care injections	938	0	938	261	0	261	2 586	126	2 460
Child sexual abuse	512	22	490	798	213	585	2 303	197	2 106

Table A5: Countries grouped by WHO region and income per capita[a] in 2004

WHO region	Income category	WHO Member States
African Region	Low and middle	Algeria, Angola, Benin, Botswana, Burkina Faso, Burundi, Cameroon, Cape Verde, Central African Republic, Chad, Comoros, Congo, Côte d'Ivoire, Democratic Republic of the Congo, Equatorial Guinea, Eritrea, Ethiopia, Gabon, Gambia, Ghana, Guinea, Guinea-Bissau, Kenya, Lesotho, Liberia, Madagascar, Malawi, Mali, Mauritania, Mauritius, Mozambique, Namibia, Niger, Nigeria, Rwanda, Sao Tome and Principe, Senegal, Seychelles, Sierra Leone, South Africa, Swaziland, Togo, Uganda, United Republic of Tanzania, Zambia, Zimbabwe
Region of the Americas	High	Bahamas, Canada, United States of America
	Low and middle	Antigua and Barbuda, Argentina, Barbados, Belize, Bolivia, Brazil, Chile, Colombia, Costa Rica, Dominica, Dominican Republic, Ecuador, El Salvador, Grenada, Guatemala, Guyana, Haiti, Honduras, Jamaica, Mexico, Nicaragua, Panama, Paraguay, Peru, Saint Kitts and Nevis, Saint Lucia, Saint Vincent and the Grenadines, Suriname, Trinidad and Tobago, Uruguay, Venezuela (Bolivarian Republic of)
Eastern Mediterranean Region	High	Bahrain, Kuwait, Qatar, Saudi Arabia, United Arab Emirates
	Low and middle	Afghanistan, Djibouti, Egypt, Iran (Islamic Republic of), Iraq, Jordan, Lebanon, Libyan Arab Jamahiriya, Morocco, Oman, Pakistan, Somalia, Sudan, Syrian Arab Republic, Tunisia, Yemen
European Region	High	Andorra, Austria, Belgium, Cyprus, Denmark, Finland, France, Germany, Greece, Iceland, Ireland, Israel, Italy, Luxembourg, Malta, Monaco, Netherlands, Norway, Portugal, San Marino, Slovenia, Spain, Sweden, Switzerland, United Kingdom
	Low and middle	Albania, Armenia, Azerbaijan, Belarus, Bosnia and Herzegovina, Bulgaria, Croatia, Czech Republic, Estonia, Georgia, Hungary, Kazakhstan, Kyrgyzstan, Latvia, Lithuania, Poland, Moldova, Romania, Russian Federation, Serbia and Montenegro, Slovakia, Tajikistan, The former Yugoslav Republic of Macedonia, Turkey, Turkmenistan, Uzbekistan, Ukraine
South-East Asia Region	Low and middle	Bangladesh, Bhutan, Democratic People's Republic of Korea, India, Indonesia, Maldives, Myanmar, Nepal, Sri Lanka, Thailand, Timor-Leste
Western Pacific Region	High	Australia, Brunei Darussalam, Japan, New Zealand, Republic of Korea, Singapore
	Low and middle	Cambodia, China, Cook Islands, Fiji, Kiribati, Lao People's Democratic Republic, Malaysia, Marshall Islands, Micronesia (Federated States of), Mongolia, Nauru, Niue, Palau, Papua New Guinea, Philippines, Samoa, Solomon Islands, Tonga, Tuvalu, Vanuatu, Viet Nam
Non-Member States or territories		American Samoa, Anguilla, Aruba, Bermuda, British Virgin Islands, Cayman Islands, Channel Islands, Faeroe Islands, Falkland Islands (Malvinas), French Guiana, French Polynesia, Gibraltar, Greenland, Guadeloupe, Guam, Holy See, Isle of Man, Liechtenstein, Martinique, Montserrat, Netherlands Antilles, New Caledonia, Northern Mariana Islands, West Bank and Gaza Strip, Pitcairn, Puerto Rico, Réunion, Saint Helena, Saint Pierre et Miquelon, Tokelau, Turks and Caicos Islands, United States Virgin Islands, Wallis and Futuna Islands, Western Sahara

[a] WHO Member States are classified as low and middle income if their 2004 gross national income per capita is less than US$ 10 066, and as high income if their 2004 gross national income per capita is US$ 10 066 or more, as estimated by the World Bank (102).

References

1. *World health report 2002. Reducing risks, promoting healthy life.* Geneva, World Health Organization, 2002.

2. *The global burden of disease: 2004 update.* Geneva, World Health Organization, 2008.

3. Commission on Social Determinants of Health. *Closing the gap in a generation: health equity through action on the social determinants of health.* Geneva, World Health Organization, 2008.

4. Rose G. Sick individuals and sick populations. *International Journal of Epidemiology*, 2001, 30:427–432.

5. Omran AR. The epidemiologic transition. A theory of the epidemiology of population change. *Milbank Memorial Fund Quarterly*, 1971, 49:509–538.

6. Mathers CD, Lopez AD, Murray CJL. The burden of disease and mortality by condition: data, methods and results for 2001. In: Lopez AD, Mathers CD, Ezzati M, Murray CJL, Jamison DT, eds. *Global burden of disease and risk factors.* New York, Oxford University Press, 2006:45–240.

7. *World health report 2004: changing history.* Geneva, World Health Organization, 2004.

8. Danaei G, Lawes CMM, Vander Hoorn S, Murray CJL, Ezzati M. Global and regional mortality from ischaemic heart disease and stroke attributable to higher-than-optimal blood glucose concentration: comparative risk assessment. *Lancet*, 2006, 368:1651–1659.

9. Black RE, Allen LH, Bhutta ZA, Caulfield LE, de Onis M, Ezzati M et al. Maternal and child undernutrition 1 — maternal and child undernutrition: global and regional exposures and health consequences. *Lancet*, 2008, 371:243–260.

10. Murray CJL, Lopez AD, Black RE, Mathers CD, Shibuya K, Ezzati M et al. Global burden of disease 2005: call for collaborators. *Lancet*, 2007, 370:109–110.

11. World Health Organization, Centers for Disease Control and Prevention. de Benoist B, McLean E, Egli I, Cogswell M, eds. *Worldwide prevalence of anaemia 1993–2005.* Geneva, World Health Organization, 2008.

12. *Global prevalence of vitamin A deficiency in populations at risk 1995–2005: WHO global database on vitamin A deficiency.* Geneva, World Health Organization, 2009.

13. *Assessment of iodine deficiency disorders and monitoring their elimination: a guide for programme managers*, 3rd ed., Geneva, World Health Organization, 2007.

14. World Health Organization, Public Health Agency of Canada. *Preventing chronic diseases: a vital investment.* Geneva, World Health Organization, 2005.

15. Ness AR, Powles JW. Fruit and vegetables, and cardiovascular disease: a review. *International Journal of Epidemiology*, 1997, 26:1–13.

16. World Cancer Research Fund, American Institute for Cancer Research. *Food, nutrition and the prevention of cancer: a global perspective.* Washington DC, American Institute for Cancer Research, 1997.

17. *WHO report on the global tobacco epidemic, 2008.* Geneva, World Health Organization, 2008.

18. *2006 World drug report.* Vienna, United Nations Office on Drugs and Crime, 2007.

19. World Health Organization, UNICEF. *Meeting the MDG drinking-water and sanitation target: the urban and rural challenge of the decade.* Geneva, World Health Organization and UNICEF Joint Monitoring Programme for Water Supply and Sanitation, 2006.

20. Ostro B. *Outdoor air pollution: assessing the environmental burden at national and local levels.* Environmental burden of disease series, No. 5. Pruss-Ustun A, Campbell-Lendrum, D, Corvalan C, Woodward A., eds. Geneva, World Health Organization, 2004.

21. Intergovernmental Panel on Climate Change. *Climate change 2007: synthesis report.* Valencia, Spain, Intergovernmental Panel on Climate Change, 2007.

22. Tennant C. Work-related stress and depressive disorders. *Journal of Psychosomatic Research*, 2001, 51:697–704.

23. Pascolini D, Smith A. Hearing impairment in 2008: a compilation of available epidemiological studies. *International Journal of Audiology*, 2009, 48:473-485.

24. *WHO guidelines for safe surgery.* Geneva, World Health Organization, 2008.

25. Andrews G, Corry J, Slade T, Issakidis C, Swanston H. Child sexual abuse. In: Ezzati M, Lopez A, Rodgers A, Murray CJL, eds. *Comparative quantification of health risks: global and regional burden of disease attributable to selected major risk factors.* Geneva, World Health Organization, 2004:1851–1940.

26. *Global status report on road safety: time for action.* Geneva, World Health Organization, 2009.

27. *World report on road traffic injury prevention.* Geneva, World Health Organization, 2004.

28. Lewington S, Whitlock G, Clarke R, Sherliker P, Emberson J, Halsey J et al. Blood cholesterol and vascular mortality by age, sex, and blood pressure: a meta-analysis of individual data from 61 prospective studies with 55,000 vascular deaths. *Lancet*, 2007, 370:1829–1839.

29. Murray CJL, Lopez AD. On the comparable quantification of health risks: lessons from the global burden of disease study. *Epidemiology*, 1999, 10:594–605.

30. Ezzati M, Lopez AD, Rodgers A, Murray CJL. *Comparative quantification of health risks: global and regional burden of disease attributable to selected major risk factors.* Geneva, World Health Organization, 2004.

31. Murray CJL, Ezzati M, Lopez AD, Rodgers A, Vander Hoorn S. Comparative quantification of health risks: conceptual framework and methodological issues. In: Ezzati M, Lopez A, Rodgers A, Murray CJL, eds. *Comparative quantification of health risks: global and regional burden of disease attributable to selected major risk factors.* Geneva, World Health Organization, 2004: 1–38.

32. Rothman KJ. Causes. *American Journal of Epidemiology*, 1976, 104:587–592.

33. Ezzati M, Vander Hoorn S, Rodgers A, Lopez AD, Mathers CD, Murray CJL et al. Estimates of global and regional potential health gains from reducing multiple major risk factors. *Lancet*, 2003, 362:271–280.

34. Wilson PW, Bozeman SR, Burton TM, Hoaglin DC, Ben Joseph R, Pashos CL. Prediction of first events of coronary heart disease and stroke with consideration of adiposity. *Circulation*, 2008, 118:124–130.

35. de Onis M, Blossner M. The World Health Organization global database on child growth and malnutrition: methodology and applications. *International Journal of Epidemiology*, 2003, 32:518–526.

36. de Onis M, Blossner M, Borghi E, Morris R, Frongillo EA. Methodology for estimating regional and global trends of child malnutrition. *International Journal of Epidemiology*, 2004, 33:1260–1270.

37. de Onis M, Garza C, Onyango AW, Martorell R. WHO child growth standards. *Acta Paediatrica Supplement*, 2006, 450:1–101.

38. *WHO child growth standards: length/height-for-age, weight-for-age, weight-for-length, weight-for-height and body mass index-for-age: methods and development.* Geneva, World Health Organization, 2006.

39. WHO Global InfoBase Team. *The SuRF report 2. Surveillance of chronic disease risk factors: country-level data and comparable estimates.* Geneva, World Health Organization, 2005.

40. Fishman SM, Caulfield LE, de Onis M, Blössner M, Hyder AA, Mullany L et al. Childhood and maternal underweight. In: Ezzati M, Lopez A, Rodgers A, Murray CJL, eds. *Comparative quantification of health risks: global and regional burden of disease attributable to selected major risk factors.* Geneva, World Health Organization, 2004:39–162.

41. Stoltzfus R, Mullany L, Black RE. Iron deficiency anaemia. In: Ezzati M, Lopez A, Rodgers A, Murray CJL, eds. *Comparative quantification of health risks: global and regional burden of disease attributable to selected major risk factors.* Geneva, World Health Organization, 2004:163–210.

42. Rice A, West KP, Black RE. Vitamin A deficiency. In: Ezzati M, Lopez A, Rodgers A, Murray CJL, eds. *Comparative quantification of health risks: global and regional burden of disease attributable to selected major risk factors. Geneva*, World Health Organization, 2004:211–256.

1

2

3

Annex A

References

43. Donath SM, Amir LH. Breastfeeding and the introduction of solids in Australian infants: data from the 2001 National Health Survey. *Australian and New Zealand Journal of Public Health*, 2005, 29:171–175.

44. *National immunization survey: provisional rates of any and exclusive breastfeeding by age among children born in 2005.* Centers for Disease Control and Prevention, Department of Health and Human Services, 2008 (http://www.cdc.gov/breastfeeding/data/NIS_data/2005/age.htm, accessed 9 July, 2008).

45. Lewington S, Clarke R, Qizilbash N, Peto R, Collins R. Age-specific relevance of usual blood pressure to vascular mortality: a meta-analysis of individual data for one million adults in 61 prospective studies. *Lancet*, 2002, 360:1903–1913.

46. Renehan AG, Tyson M, Egger M, Heller RF, Zwahlen M. Body-mass index and incidence of cancer: a systematic review and meta-analysis of prospective observational studies. *Lancet*, 2008, 371:569–578.

47. Ni MC, Rodgers A, Pan WH, Gu DF, Woodward M. Body mass index and cardiovascular disease in the Asia–Pacific Region: an overview of 33 cohorts involving 310 000 participants. *International Journal of Epidemiology*, 2004, 33:751–758.

48. James WPT, Jackson-Leach R, Ni Mhurchu C, Kalamara E, Shayeghi M, Rigby NJ et al. Overweight and obesity (high body mass index). In: Ezzati M, Lopez A, Rodgers A, Murray CJL, eds. *Comparative quantification of health risks: global and regional burden of disease attributable to selected major risk factors.* Geneva, World Health Organization, 2004:959–1108.

49. Lock K, Pomerleau J, Causer L, McKee M. Low fruit and vegetable consumption. In: Ezzati M, Lopez AD, Rodgers A, Murray CJL, eds. *Comparative quantification of health risks: global and regional burden of disease attributable to selected major risk factors.* Geneva, World Health Organization, 2004:597–728.

50. Danaei G, Ding E, Taylor B, Mozaffarian D, Rehm J, Murray CJL et al. Mortality effects of lifestyle, dietary, and metabolic risk factors in the United States: comparative risk assessment. *PLoS Medicine*, 2009, 6(4):e1000058.

51. Dauchet L, Amouyel P, Hercberg S, Dallongeville J. Fruit and vegetable consumption and risk of coronary heart disease: a meta-analysis of cohort studies. *Journal of Nutrition*, 2006, 136:2588–2593.

52. Dauchet L, Amouyel P, Dallongeville J. Fruit and vegetable consumption and risk of stroke: a meta-analysis of cohort studies. *Neurology*, 2005, 65:1193–1197.

53. Boeing H, Dietrich T, Hoffmann K, Pischon T, Ferrari P, Lahmann PH et al. Intake of fruits and vegetables and risk of cancer of the upper aero-digestive tract: the prospective EPIC-study. *Cancer Causes and Control*, 2006, 17:957–969.

54. Bull FC, Armstrong TP, Dixon TD, Ham S, Neiman A, Pratt M. Physical inactivity. In: Ezzati M, Lopez A, Rodgers A, Murray CJL, eds. *Comparative quantification of health risks: global and regional burden of disease attributable to selected major risk factors.* Geneva, World Health Organization, 2004.

55. Begg S, Vos T, Barker B, Stevenson C, Stanley L, Lopez A. *The burden of disease and injury in Australia 2003.* Canberra, Australian Institute of Health and Welfare, 2007.

56. *Stepwise approach to surveillance (STEPS).* World Health Organization, 2008 (http://www.who.int/chp/steps/en/, accessed 8 July 2009).

57. Lawes CM, Parag V, Bennett DA, Suh I, Lam TH, Whitlock G et al. Blood glucose and risk of cardiovascular disease in the Asia Pacific region. *Diabetes Care*, 2004, 27:2836–2842.

58. Slaymaker E, Walker N, Zaba B, Collumbien M. Unsafe sex. In: Ezzati M, Lopez A, Rodgers A, Murray CJL, eds. *Comparative quantification of health risks: global and regional burden of disease attributable to selected major risk factors.* Geneva, World Health Organization, 2004:1177–1255.

59. UNAIDS, World Health Organization. *AIDS epidemic update: December 2003.* Geneva, UNAIDS, 2003.

60. UNAIDS. *2004 report on the global AIDS epidemic.* Geneva, UNAIDS, 2004.

61. UNAIDS, World Health Organization. *AIDS epidemic update: December 2005.* Geneva, UNAIDS, 2005.

62. UNAIDS, World Health Organization. *AIDS epidemic update: December 2006.* Geneva, UNAIDS, 2006.

63. UNAIDS, World Health Organization. *AIDS epidemic update: December 2007.* Geneva, UNAIDS, 2007.

64. Steinbrook R. HIV in India—a complex epidemic. *New England Journal of Medicine*, 2007, 356:1089–1093.

65. Walboomers JM, Jacobs MV, Manos MM, Bosch FX, Kummer JA, Shah KV et al. Human papillomavirus is a necessary cause of invasive cervical cancer worldwide. *Journal of Pathology*, 1999, 189:12–19.

66. Collumbien M, Gerressu M, Cleland J. Non-use and use of ineffective methods of contraception. In: Ezzati M, Lopez A, Rodgers A, Murray CJL, eds. *Comparative quantification of health risks: global and regional burden of disease attributable to selected major risk factors.* Geneva, World Health Organization, 2004:1255–1319.

67. Population Division, UN Department of Economic and Social Affairs. *World contraceptive use 2007.* New York, United Nations, 2008.

68. Peto R, Lopez AD, Boreham J, Thun M, Heath C Jr. Mortality from tobacco in developed countries: indirect estimation from national vital statistics. *Lancet*, 1992, 339:1268–1278.

69. Thun MJ, Apicella LF, Henley SJ. Smoking vs other risk factors as the cause of smoking-attributable deaths: confounding in the courtroom. *Journal of the American Medical Association*, 2000, 284:706–712.

70. International Institute for Population Sciences, World Health Organization. *World Health Survey 2003, India.* Mumbai, International Institute for Population Sciences, 2006 (http://www.who.int/healthinfo/survey/whs_hspa_book.pdf, accessed 8 July, 2009).

71. Ezzati M, Henley SJ, Lopez AD, Thun MJ. Role of smoking in global and regional cancer epidemiology: current patterns and data needs. *International Journal of Cancer*, 2005, 116:963–971.

72. Ezzati M, Henley SJ, Thun MJ, Lopez AD. Role of smoking in global and regional cardiovascular mortality. *Circulation*, 2005, 112:489–497.

73. Lin HH, Ezzati M, Murray M. Tobacco smoke, indoor air pollution and tuberculosis: a systematic review and meta-analysis. *PLoS Medicine*, 2007, 4:e20.

74. Rao DN, Ganesh B, Rao RS, Desai PB. Risk assessment of tobacco, alcohol and diet in oral cancer—a case-control study. *International Journal of Cancer*, 1994, 58:469–473.

75. Kehoe T, Rehm J, Chatterji S. *Global burden of alcohol use disorders in the year 2004.* Report prepared for WHO. Zurich, Switzerland, WHO Collaboration Centre at the Research Centre for Public Health and Addiction, 2007.

76. Rehm J, Room R, Monteiro M, Gmel G, Graham K, Rehn N et al. Alcohol use. In: Ezzati M, Lopez A, Rodgers A, Murray CJL, eds. *Comparative quantification of health risks: global and regional burden of disease attributable to selected major risk factors.* Geneva, World Health Organization, 2004: 959–1108.

77. Rehm J, Mathers CD, Patra J, Thavorncharoensap M, Teerawattananon Y. Global burden of disease and injury and economic cost attributable to alcohol use and alcohol-use disorders. *Lancet*, 2009, 373(9682):2223–2233.

78. Baan R, Straif K, Grosse Y, Secretan B, El GF, Bouvard V et al. Carcinogenicity of some aromatic amines, organic dyes, and related exposures. *Lancet Oncology*, 2008, 9:322–323.

79. Degenhardt L, Hall W, Warner-Smith M, Lynskey M. Illicit drugs. In: Ezzati M, Lopez A, Rodgers A, Murray CJL, eds. *Comparative quantification of health risks: global and regional burden of disease attributable to selected major risk factors.* Geneva, World Health Organization, 2003.

80. Pruss-Ustun A, Kay D, Fewtrell L, Bartram J. Unsafe water, sanitation and hygiene. In: Ezzati M, Lopez A, Rodgers A, Murray CJL, eds. *Comparative quantification of health risks: global and regional burden of disease attributable to selected major risk factors.* Geneva, World Health Organization, 2004: 1321–1352.

81. Cohen A, Anderson H, Ostro B, Pandey K, Krzyzanowski M, Kunzli N et al. Urban air pollution. In: Ezzati M, Lopez A, Rodgers A, Murray CJL, eds. *Comparative quantification of health risks: global and regional burden of disease attributable to selected major risk factors.* Geneva, World Health Organization, 2004:1353–1433.

82. European Environment Information and Observation Network. *European air quality database.* European Environmental Agency, 2009 (http://air-climate.eionet.europa.eu/databases/airbase/, accessed 8 July, 2009).

83. *Indoor air pollution: national burden of disease.* Geneva, World Health Organization, 2007 (http://www.who.int/indoorair/publications/indoor_air_national_burden_estimate_revised.pdf, accessed 8 July, 2009).

84. Smith K, Mehta S, Maeusezahl-Feuz M. Indoor air pollution from household use of solid fuels. In: Ezzati M, Lopez A, Rodgers A, Murray CJL, eds. *Comparative quantification of health risks: global and regional burden of disease attributable to selected major risk factors.* Geneva, World Health Organization, 2004:1435–1493.

85. Pruss-Ustun A, Fewtrell L, Landrigan PJ, Ayuso-Mateos JL. Lead exposure. In: Ezzati M, Lopez A, Rodgers A, Murray CJL, eds. *Comparative quantification of health risks: global and regional burden of disease attributable to selected major risk factors.* Geneva, World Health Organization, 2004:1495–1542.

86. McMichael AJ, Campbell-Lendrum D, Kovats S, Edwards S, Wilkinson P, Wilson T et al. Global Climate Change. In: Ezzati M, Lopez A, Rodgers A, Murray CJL, eds. *Comparative quantification of health risks: global and regional burden of disease attributable to selected major risk factors.* Geneva, World Health Organization, 2004:1543–1650.

87. Concha-Barrientos M, Nelson DI, Driscoll T, Steenland NK, Punnett L, Fingerhut MA et al. Selected occupational risks. In: Ezzati M, Lopez A, Rodgers A, Murray CJL, eds. *Comparative quantification of health risks: global and regional burden of disease attributable to selected major risk factors.* Geneva, World Health Organization, 2004:1652–1801.

88. Driscoll T, Nelson DI, Steenland K, Leigh J, Concha-Barrientos M, Fingerhut M et al. The global burden of disease due to occupational carcinogens. *American Journal of Industrial Medicine,* 2005, 48:419–431.

89. Driscoll T, Nelson DI, Steenland K, Leigh J, Concha-Barrientos M, Fingerhut M et al. The global burden of non-malignant respiratory disease due to occupational airborne exposures. *American Journal of Industrial Medicine,* 2005, 48:432–445.

90. Hauri AM, Gregory I, Armstrong L, Hutin YJF. Contaminated injections in health care settings. In: Ezzati M, Lopez A, Rodgers A, Murray CJL, eds. *Comparative quantification of health risks: global and regional burden of disease attributable to selected major risk factors.* Geneva, World Health Organization, 2004: 1803–1850.

1

2

3

Annex A

References

91. Hauri AM, Armstrong GL, Hutin YJF. The global burden of disease attributable to contaminated injections given in health care settings. *International Journal of STD AIDS*, 2004, 15:7–16.

92. Baggaley RF, Boily MC, White RG, Alary M. Risk of HIV-1 transmission for parenteral exposure and blood transfusion: a systematic review and meta-analysis. *AIDS*, 2006, 20:805–812.

93. Schmid GP, Buve A, Mugyenyi P, Garnett GP, Hayes RJ, Williams BG et al. Transmission of HIV-1 infection in sub-Saharan Africa and effect of elimination of unsafe injections. *Lancet*, 2004, 363:482–488.

94. White RG, Ben SC, Kedhar A, Orroth KK, Biraro S, Baggaley RF et al. Quantifying HIV-1 transmission due to contaminated injections. *Proceedings of the National Academy of Science of the United States of America*, 2007, 104:9794–9799.

95. National AIDS Control Organization. *UNGASS country progress report 2008: India.* Ministry of Health and Family Welfare, Government of India, 2008.

96. UNAIDS, World Health Organization. *Resource needs for AIDS in low- and middle-income countries: estimation process and methods. Methodological annex II: revised projections of the number of people in need of ART.* Geneva, UNAIDS, 2007.

97. *Time from HIV-1 seroconversion to AIDS and death before widespread use of highly-active antiretroviral therapy: a collaborative re-analysis.* Collaborative Group on AIDS Incubation and HIV Survival including the CASCADE EU Concerted Action. Concerted Action on SeroConversion to AIDS and Death in Europe. *Lancet*, 2000, 355:1131–1137.

98. Gouws E, White PJ, Stover J, Brown T. Short term estimates of adult HIV incidence by mode of transmission: Kenya and Thailand as examples. *Sexually Transmitted Infections*, 2006, 82:iii51–iii55.

99. Kiwanuka N, Gray RH, Serwadda D, Li X, Sewankambo NK, Kigozi G et al. The incidence of HIV-1 associated with injections and transfusions in a prospective cohort, Rakai, Uganda. *AIDS*, 2004, 18:342–344.

100. Parkin DM. The global health burden of infection-associated cancers in the year 2002. *International Journal of Cancer*, 2006, 118:3030–3044.

101. Perz JF, Armstrong GL, Farrington LA, Hutin YJ, Bell BP. The contributions of hepatitis B virus and hepatitis C virus infections to cirrhosis and primary liver cancer worldwide. *Journal of Hepatology*, 2006, 45:529–38.

102. *World development report 2004: equity and development.* Washington DC, The World Bank, 2006.